Virginia Pierce

MALAWI MOONSMOKE

Changing a Part of Our World -- One Life at a Time

Because you also care for the little ones.

BEE BIGGS-JARRELL

Bee Biggs-Jarrell

Outskirts Press, Inc.
Denver, Colorado

beeken90@gmail

The opinions expressed in this manuscript are solely the opinions of the author and do not represent the opinions or thoughts of the publisher. The author represents and warrants that s/he either owns or has the legal right to publish all material in this book. If you believe this to be incorrect, contact the publisher through its website at www.outskirtspress.com.

Malawi Moonsmoke
Changing a Part of Our World -- One Life at a Time
All Rights Reserved
Copyright © 2006 Bee Biggs-Jarrell
Cover Image © 2006 JupiterImages Corporation
All Rights Reserved. Used With Permission.

This book may not be reproduced, transmitted, or stored in whole or in part by any means, including graphic, electronic, or mechanical without the express written consent of the publisher except in the case of brief quotations embodied in critical articles and reviews.

Outskirts Press
http://www.outskirtspress.com

ISBN-10: 1-59800-342-9
ISBN-13: 978-1-59800-342-0

Library of Congress Control Number: 2006926563

Outskirts Press and the "OP" logo are trademarks belonging to Outskirts Press, Inc.

Printed in the United States of America

MALAWI MOONSMOKE

An Anthology
Of
Interdenominational Mission Life in Malawi

By

Bee Biggs-Jarrell, RN, BSN, MPA

Volunteer in Public Health Service for the Development of Malawi

Changing Our World, One Life at a Time
With
Adventist Development and Relief Agency (ADRA)
In partnership with Nsanje District, Malawi Village Churches
Kalemba Parish, Catholic Clinic
Trinity Hospital Parish, Catholic
Bangula Central Church of Africa, Presbyterian
Bangula Anglicans
Bangula Episcopal Women's Group
Chideu Village Church of God
Malawi Ministry of Health

Dedication

This book is dedicated to...

those committed Malawian Health Surveillance Assistants, their professional leaders in service on both the East and West Banks of the giant Shire River, who by their service, helped take religious denominational walls down. They gave all they had to follow the way of Jesus Christ in serving their people and their nation to help cleanse the atmosphere of the toxic "moon smoke" and show a better way of life for families now and in the future.

Acknowledgments

During the past thirteen years since we first returned from our life-changing experience of service in the African nation of Malawi, *Moonsmoke* has bubbled up through my consciousness and my computer in bits and pieces as time and as active memory permitted. I have told many of these stories in University classrooms, elementary schools, churches, women's groups and around campfires. They were illustrated with the lively video segments we made during our two-year journey there and back. Because of my Heavenly Father's guiding hand, and the loving support from many friends and family members, I am, at last, seeing the anthology in print. I extend my deepest appreciation to them all.

It was my God's guidance that enabled my academic, experiential, and spiritual development as preparation for Malawi years before I even dreamed of going there. I stand in awe of how He entrusted the gentle lives of hundreds of villagers into my care. Finally, I believe it is God's soft nudging that ultimately compelled me to write these stories. He has my highest praise!

To my husband, Ken, who dared to love me enough to

leave all that was familiar and join me, first in commitment to the vision of Christian service, then in love, marriage and transplantation to the third world. Ken you were my coach in critiquing and affirming my project leadership then, and now. You snapped the photos and captured the videos that enrich the memories and these stories. You gave me encouragement to keep on during the rough days, and the freedom to change course during the project. You transferred your wisdom and knowledge of machinery to people who had never held a wrench in their hands. Your teaching kept the project motor vehicles running and the bicycles in repair! Your support during the years since the Malawi experience enabled the book to emerge. During recent years that took us both through several personal detours in medical diagnoses and critical surgeries; you kept me adding notes toward the publication of this book.

To my children and grandchildren, who patiently listened to the stories and believed that Grandma Bee would eventually get *Moonsmoke* into print, you were often an inspiration to me.

To dear friend and colleague, Marge Wilcox who read and reread these stories many times, provided priceless feedback, and consistent support and improvement for the book project. Your professional writer and teacher's background helped enliven word pictures, amplified the rich range of experiential emotions I tried to depict, and you significantly enriched the fiber of the stories' woven fabric.

To Lois Moore, who with her husband Marvin, came to love the people of Malawi so much through our verbal pictures, that they helped to fund construction of the Mphonde Village Church to seat over 500 people, where all are welcome who seek to know Jesus Christ as their Savior. Mphonde serves a huge catchment area where there had been no church of any denomination previously. Lois and Marvin also provided valuable, in-depth manuscript review and suggestions. Thank you!

To the hundreds of people with whom we worked, prayed, taught, and, yes...even played, during those two years in Malawi. Some of your names were not used at all; others names have been changed; still others names are used confidently that we have your permission to do so. You enriched our lives as you taught us patiently how to live, love and be effective within the Malawi culture.

I extend deepest appreciation to those dear friends who read any of the sequence of manuscripts, and offered encouragement and suggestions for editing and improving the work. Your contributions are invaluable! Michelle Maxwell, Cathy McCrea, Marge Wagner, Patricia Young, and Judy Murray.

Table of Contents

CHAPTER 1

Out of the Gloom

Healing for Grief and Loss

I awakened suddenly to the silent darkness, in my room. Almost palpable darkness engulfed me; out of my window, I couldn't see the stars, or any moon. Why was my room so silent? and the place beside me so cold? -- emptiness. My hand reached across the smooth sheet to find my husband of thirty-six years. He was not there. He had been so sick the past few days. The nurse within me prompted with an order, "Get up, and see if he is all right!" Still not fully awake, my feet found the floor. My stirring mind questioned, "Why is he out of bed with no light on?" With a touch, light flooded my room and I became fully awake.

He was not there. He was not in the house. A chill swept over my trembling body as awareness struck me and tears splashed down my face. The empty place beside me would always be empty, I thought. My lover and wonderful husband of 36 years, Cree, had died a month earlier. Quietly, at peace with himself and his God, his great heart of love had pumped most of his life-blood out through a broken artery serving the kidney, and with not enough to pump, his heart had stopped.

In the deep darkness of the night, that agonizing scene ripped fiercely through my tired mind once again. There were waves of guilt and unanswerable questions. Had I been wrong to tell the doctors to "let him go" without opening the belly and trying to patch the leak? Was his great loss to me and our children my fault for not demanding heroic efforts at that time?

The ache inside me seemed to squeeze out my breath. At two o'clock in the morning, there was just one thing to do. I turned out the light and took my aching body, mind, and spirit back to the very cold bed. In the darkness and pain, I cried out to my God, "Why have you forsaken me?" Even as I spoke, I remembered that His Son had uttered those same words in enormously greater anguish than mine, as He died for me on the cross. At that moment, I began to realize as never before, something of Jesus Christ's great love and loss on my account. As I prayed, the Spirit of Christ was very near, whispering His promises to my hurting soul. "I will never leave you or forsake you," "My peace I give unto you", "Be of good cheer, for I have overcome...." I felt a new and closer relationship beginning with my Lord.

Companionship with my earthly lover and best friend was lost; but softly and gradually filling that aching, ugly hole in my heart came Jesus, Himself. I began to "practice the presence of God" whenever my overwhelming sense of loss cast dark shadows on me. More than ever, I talked to Him and invited Him into my deepest consciousness, as I continued my responsible Public Health Administration work in Idaho State Government, and as I managed my home, making decisions alone as I had never done before. And He always spoke back to me with words of encouragement -- or little miracles -- or special protection when driving my mountain roads -- and keeping me from the harm of a high-powered sniper's bullet through my living room window.

The sniper incident occurred in the wee hours of the morning after my birthday. The house was full of my grown children and several grandchildren. I remember that as I retired, I had marveled at the bright trail of moonlight that bathed our home. It had been a lovely day and it was a beautiful night without a cloud and a full moon. Suddenly I was awakened by the explosive "POW" of a high-powered gunshot. My first thought was, "Ooh, that is a gunshot and it comes from too close by!" But before I could think again another shot rang out, and another, and then "POW! CRASH! Clink, clink" as the bullet came through my highest living room window. As the shots continued rapidly, I sent a thought prayer, "Lord, please stop that gunman and keep us safe!"

Even with all the noise, my children and grandchildren slept on, while I called out to my oldest son, "Jay, we have taken a bullet!" He was at my bedside immediately. As I stood up, glass fragments fell from my hair. We found the bedside flashlight and dialed the sheriff's number, who told us not to turn on any lights and that he would be there in ten minutes. When the sheriff arrived, we turned on all the lights, finding shattered glass everywhere, even imbedded in the tabletop and the wall. We found the slug in the ceiling.

As we inspected the damage, a neighbor telephoned, seeing our lights, to ask if that gunman hit us. She described what she had heard and seen in the full moonlight -- a person with a pickup truck, taking aim across his open door. Suddenly there was no more moonlight for me. I felt cold chills. Someone hated me, -- who, and why? Glass shards were imbedded in the walls, the furniture and throughout the carpet. We drew close together, five adults and three children, praying and thanking God that none of us had been hurt and asking Him to take care of the person with that gun. The sheriff arrived to find us praying.

Law enforcement authorities' theories were developed and a full investigation was undertaken, but not enough evidence was found to charge anyone with this cowardly act that was obviously intended to frighten me and my family. As a public health official, I had recently denied a license to a man who had been abusing the elderly in his care. Was this his "get even" move? A neighbor dropped in the next morning and callously insinuated to me that someone was upset with my politics since I had publicly supported the Idaho Governor as he sought a national political office. Another theory was that perhaps someone was trying to frighten me into fleeing my home in fear and possibly selling it for less than it was worth.

The sheriff instructed me, "Young lady," he said, "you get a handgun and learn how to use it." My military son, Mark, was right there and chimed in, "Sure, I'll teach her how to use it. She was a crack-shot with my 22 the other day." I listened, but the Holy Spirit whispered clearly to me, and that night I went to the Holy Scripture. Looking up every reference on fear and then every reference on peace, I claimed the peace promises and declined the opportunity to own or use a handgun. It took weeks to have my custom-made window replaced, and I was almost sad when it was finished, because it had given me many opportunities to witness for my Jesus and His dependable protection in every circumstance.

All the time, He was very close to me, reassuring me, and bringing me peace. Joshua 1:9 played over and over in my mind. "Have I not commanded you? Be strong and courageous. Do not be terrified; do not be discouraged, for the Lord your God will be with you wherever you go."Friends and family took on new meaning for me at this time. Our three grown sons and a daughter had celebrated their precious dad's life in a memorial ceremony. In their tender and solicitous attitudes toward me and my needs, it seemed that they tried to do and be everything to me, to be sure that I could manage on my own. I enjoyed being wrapped up in their love My new emotional fragility was a bit of surprise to me and to many others, since an uncommon psychic strength had seemed to serve me well through many other crises in my life. I suppose that age had something to do with this fragility, too -- I was well past sixty years old.

What began as the emotional pain of great loss, reached further with strong tentacles to become physical pain. Very real in its nature, this pain unaccountably involved just the left side of my body, including the left arm, left chest wall, searing my left hip and clutching my entire left leg. My physician prescribed pain medicine when aspirin and ibuprofen had no effect. But the pain never left me. Then my best friend, Jesus, came with a miracle of healing and changed everything!

It was on the shores of Payette Lake in central Idaho where I went to pray with some other Christian women just two months after Cree died. On the first night of the retreat, I was prompted by the Holy Spirit to share my physical pain experience with these wonderful women and ask for their prayers. Along with many other petitions, my request ascended on the breeze from beneath the lakeshore pines, as we joined in prayer that night. We continued in study, prayer, and praise for two days. On the second day, I awakened to a full moon casting its shimmering pathway across the waters of the lake. I had gone to sleep with an aching body and a longing heart, but in this early hour of the morning, I suddenly was free! Free of the body pain, free of the anguish, and I felt a healing warmth flood my body, just as though I had been wrapped in a heated blanket. Jesus was reaching down and touching me just then. He touched me and I knew it was my special miracle from Him! I silently wept for joy and offered my prayer of appreciation, for I knew that He indeed, reached through time and space and touched me in this beautiful moment, in the misty light of the mountain moon. Jesus touched me!

As a golden dawn descended on the silence and beauty of a still sleeping mountain camp, I quietly dressed and slipped out of the dormitory, visualizing Jesus at my side, rejoicing with me, taking my left hand in His, giving my hand a squeeze. And there was no more pain; only warmth, vitality and an indescribable joy sweeping over me. Together, with these wonderful praying women, Jesus and I had become a miracle! Tears of gratitude and joy rolled down my cheeks. I did not want the moment to end. But, also, I felt I could not wait to tell my very personal miracle of healing to the women who had been praying. When I told them, almost two-hundred women rejoiced, praised God and sang and prayed with me that morning. Everything changed for me that day with Jesus!

My professional work took on a new focus. And I had an amazing new vitality, new love and joy flowed through me that, to me, was quietly astounding. Worries left me; instead, creativity flowed. It was as though His Spirit was saying to me: "Don't waste your time wondering about your problems. My grace is sufficient for you, so let's figure out together what to do about this, or that, very real concern." Always, with study, prayer, and counsel from good friend or family members, solutions for life's very real issues came. My trust in God was growing!

Relationships that had seemed strained over little disagreements were mended and began to flourish. I remember a neighbor who had exhibited open jealousy toward me, the new widow, who seemed to pose a threat to her marriage. It was after church worship services one Sabbath in December, when my pastor reached out and gave me a "holy hug." This dear Christian neighbor who heretofore seemed to share my grief and loss of my husband (and her friend), rushed to my side, emphatically whispering in a rasping sound, "This hugging in the church has got to STOP!" I felt an icy cold chill sweep down over my heart. I ran to my son's car and wept and wept. When the children and grandchildren came to the car for the drive home, I was still weeping uncontrollably. They tried to console me, but I couldn't even tell them what had brought on this explosion of grief.

Trying to cheer me up, the children suggested that we pack a snow picnic and head for a spot high in the white hills. But I declined, saying that I felt I needed to be alone in prayer. Needless to say, I just knelt and prayed most of the afternoon. At first, as I poured out my stricken, rejected heart to Jesus, I could think of no reason for my neighbor's behavior. But as I took it to Jesus, He showed me understanding and forgiveness for her attitude. Suddenly I saw that some of my actions since becoming a widow may have posed a threat to her marriage. Her husband, an elder in our church, had hugged me on numerous occasions, offering kind, supportive help, grieving with me, because my husband had been his friend, too. I began to see how my closeness to her husband might have made her feel very insecure, and my actions had become a stumbling block for her.

Jesus guided me right that afternoon to write both of them a note asking that the husband not hug me anymore, even in friendship, and also asking forgiveness for my "stumbling block" behavior. I went to their door to deliver the note, but they were not at home, so I tucked it securely into the door and left it, somewhat relieved that I didn't need to see them in person just yet. They never brought up the note or the incident, but there was no more hugging. Years later, this Sister in the Lord and I wept in each others arms in mutual forgiveness, understanding and sisterly love, just four weeks before she died. From this delicate experience, I learned that even a "holy hug" could be a stumbling block to some others who do not feel the freedom to give or take such touching. And I learned to be more careful of others' personal space and preferences, especially when a handshake would do!

As I accomplished some major work objectives and leadership within the Idaho Division of Health, I began to think about what might lie ahead. Retirement was not far away. What does a healthy, creative, born again retiree do for the Lord? A recurring thought from the Holy Scriptures kept playing each time I thought of retirement from the workaday world. "...Whatever you did for one of the least of these brothers of mine, you did for me." (Matthew 25:40, last part). So, I just asked Him, "Jesus, who are the least? In this land of plenty, where are the least? How do I use all the gifts you have given me, to find and serve the least?" His answer again, was clear.

"Child of mine, bloom right here where I have planted you. If you feel hemmed in as a government worker, retire early. Teach what you have learned. Teach the parents about their children. Teach about my love in your community, church, and Sabbath School. Continue to be faithful in a few little things, and let me surprise you with what I will do with you. Whatever happens, you know that you are not alone. I am with you right into the uttermost parts of the earth."

My heart was stirred with this new vision. Retire now! And teach! He gave me the gifts and the preparation, and He will be with me as I use the gifts in new ways! Wow! But what is this about the "uttermost parts of the earth"? He seemed to be saying to me: "Stay busy, teaching the least of these (the children) because I will take you to the uttermost parts of the earth."

"Okay, Lord," I said, "I'll do it." Within the second year of widowhood, I retired and obtained a grant to teach high-risk parents positive new parenting skills. The local Magistrate judge in my mountain area assisted in designing the course, and assigned the parents to attend the classes when their children manifested delinquent behavior. The grant paid for class materials and my expenses, so that the parents (most of them very poor), could attend without cost, since their attendance was mandated by the court. I saw lives changed for the better as these parents learned to accept themselves and as they took on new attitudes and new skills in guiding and disciplining their children. This course was in demand in several communities across southern Idaho, and I was free to go where I was needed. I enjoyed being my own boss, taking the Active Parenting classes wherever I was invited and finding a deep, new friendship with Patricia the local Magistrate.

A vacation trip took me to visit friends and relatives on the eastern coast of the United States. While planning the trip, Jesus whispered to me, "Think about international service for me, and while you are in Washington, DC, stop in at the world headquarters of your church and offer your gifts in volunteer service." I was astonished at the thought! How could I go away from home where I am known and doors to my service are already opened? What would I do about my home, my dog, and my cat? Jesus' answer came, "I have taught you not to worry, so just continue to trust me. This is another door that could open, so you need to at least knock on the door."

So knock I did. Surprisingly, the chief church health official seemed unable to believe that I was volunteering. A physician about my age, he seemed to speak patronizingly to me, cajoling me, toying with my idea of being helpful with health needs anywhere in the world. Finally, he told me that he was just so sorry, there were no jobs available at this time. I was amazed that this official did not seem to know what I was talking about when I said I wanted to volunteer to serve the poorest of the poor. "The least of these, somewhere in the world." On the way out of the office building, a receptionist sensed my disappointment in not being immediately able to "sign up," and she handed me a brochure from another part of the church bureaucracy that placed volunteers in service, in countries around the world. Right away, I completed the information and left my "sign up" form in Washington, DC.

The Good Ol' Boys

During this third year of widowhood, my devotional time was centered mainly on studies on effectual prayer and the power of the Holy Spirit. I was impressed to lead a women's prayer group, which met every Monday morning at 6:30 for a bit of breakfast, sharing, and prayer. We were a very mutually satisfying support group and found that in praying together there was power, not only to effect the changes in our lives that we needed, but also dynamic, intercessory power for others. It was in this group that I learned from studying What Happens When Women Pray by Evelyn Christenson, to pray and really mean it: "Father, I want your will in **every area** of my life including my work, my home, my health, my children, my loved ones, and my service for you. Amen."

Lloyd John Ogilvie's writings also influenced my prayer life as I came to understand that every one of my prayers is initiated in the mind of God. He gives me the issues and He gives me the answers. Often I would just feel the need to talk with God, -- it didn't matter where I was, and my prayer would be, "So, what did you want to talk to me about, Lord?" And, always he brought an important issue to my mind for our consideration together.

From John L. Shuler's book, The Holy Spirit, Your Best Helper, came the Biblical reassurance that:

The "fellowship with the Spirit" (Philippians 2:1) and the "fellowship of the Holy Spirit" (2 Corinthians 13:14) provide for believers a relationship similar to that which Jesus had with His Father. (John 6:57 and 14:10). It constitutes the closest possible union and companionship you can have with your Savior. It is closer and sweeter than the fellowship that can exist between dearest friends or even husband and wife.

Again, WOW! God let me see it in black and white print so that I would know for certain that this was what He was giving to me in my time of loss. I could not stay quiet about it! Whenever I was given the opening, I would share this JOY that He had brought to me. Living moment by moment with him and I imagine ten thousand angels, there was never a dull moment, and hasn't been to this day!!

One wintry day I was at my little breakfast table, writing letters to my children, when I noticed a lone coyote across the snowy canyon, high on the bluff, and I began to fantasize about this solitary animal, and I wrote:

> Her lonely quest was in the wintertime, and in the winter season of her life. Two winters had passed since she'd lost her mate to the Trapper.
>
> As she trudged through the deep snow, she stopped often to catch her breath. It was not always this difficult, and at times her heart now pounded and her chest heaved with the effort. Always listening and sniffing the air, she remembered the bright, warm years spent with him.
>
> He was elegant in build and movement; always he brought the results of his hunt to her first. He chose her company over that of the other males, saw that their mountain den was safe and secure, and he went out of his way to be playful with her and to please her.
>
> Together they raised their young -- healthy, playful challenges that came along regularly in the springtime of their lives. How they worked together to teach them the skills that they would need! They would need skills, not

just to survive, but skills to thrive in their times: how, whom and what senses to trust; being part of, and loyal to the family, and ultimately independence and living free!

But, now, as the drifts grew deeper, she wondered if she'd see those young ones again. They had their own mates and their own young. For friends, there were a few older females like herself -- but they often seemed cranky, wanting to be left alone, and very few seemed to have her zest for life -- And there were even fewer males.

As she raised her head to fresh pine smells, she remembered his scent, and how they had snuggled for warmth and safety. And her great heart nearly burst with longing for his nose nuzzling and his proud and gentle caresses.

Finding food in the snow seemed more of an ordeal this winter than last. Or was she slower, or the food just more scarce? Hunting together had been so easy, so much fun and how they had enjoyed sharing their bounty.

Glancing upward, she noticed a pair of bald eagles soaring on the wind in their quest for food. They seemed not to notice her, but, she thought, "Such sweet companionship," as the eagles soared out of sight.

She pushed on -- up the steep, rocky exposed south face of the mountain to territory she knew little about. Just as darkness came and the crystal cold moon rose, she found food, enough to sustain her while she sought shelter for the night. The rocky face glistened in the moonlight, except for one black shadow. It might be shelter. She stood, trembling with exhaustion, then slowly moved toward the dark space. Soft, reflected light from a million snow crystals showed an open, covered cleft in the rock. And there in that reflected light stood a great, graying, and shaggy male of her kind. He yelped and whined as if to question. She showed no fear and tentatively, came slowly toward him. She felt the great shuddering thrill of him as he circled her once, -- and the nose nuzzling began.

As I pondered this fantasy, I knew that it must be an allegory to my own life and loss experience. I had been studying everything I could find in respectable literature on the phenomenon of grief, and how one can grow from a healthy grief experience. This little fantasy (I didn't dare to call it a vision!) was a delightful treasure for me to ponder, then and is even now.

Then, the telephone began to ring and there were knocks on my social door from dear and wonderful old friends -- or friends of friends -- the "good ol' boys" from college and even high school days. Their wives had either died prematurely or there had been a divorce. I said to my Lord, "Are you bringing these men into my life in order for me to consider another marriage?" The answer was very clear. I had prayed the prayer, wanting His will in every aspect of my life. So after the initial surprise and bewilderment, I began to enjoy the attention. There were special little dinners, a picnic in the park, and a walk in the Julia Davis Rose Garden, which proved to be fatal for this suitor after he said to this rose lover that he just hates roses because they are so much work. That put an end to any further responses from me to his attentions.

One old friend attended church with me, and I learned later that the talk went around that this would be the man for Bee! But he failed my tests two ways in that he had many criticisms about the house that was my home, built by Cree and me, and furthermore, he did not enjoy climbing

"Sunshine Mountain," a gentle butte that rises out of my south yard. How could anyone not enjoy hiking this little hill?

Another friend of a friend was overly retired -- I thought, "just plain tired," and he could not understand why I would not enjoy sitting in twin rockers watching all his favorite television shows! The best looking, and seemingly most active of these good ol' boys, wanted sex today and then we can discuss a longer term relationship -- and he at that time was a missionary to Mexico!

After providing a worship service for a Christian Singles Ministry at Camp Mivoden in northern Idaho, I joined up. This is a group that provides a ministry to singles, in every sense of the word. From fellowshipping with them, I found new friends, some more good ol' boys! and a new satisfaction in being single in my walk with God's children.

Reflecting upon the interesting dynamics of my good ol' boys experiences, I remember telling God one day that if those fellows and those experiences were all that He had for me, please don't waste my time anymore. Besides, if He wanted me in some foreign country ministering to His little ones, I asked Him, "Wouldn't a husband just be extra baggage? But, nevertheless," I added, "Thy will be done in my life!"

Then came another September Christian Women's Retreat, the same retreat where my major miracle of healing had happened three years before. The speaker for the weekend suggested that each woman choose one issue on which to focus for the session and make that the center of her prayer. I remember almost the exact wording that I began to pray about, over and over again that weekend:

> Dear Father, please show me how you want me to live -- single or remarried -- and where you want me to go in the "uttermost parts of the earth" to serve the "least of them."

There was no handwriting on the wall for me; no

miraculous answer for me to share with my prayer partners this time. I went home to Clifcrest still praying that prayer on a daily basis.

Beginning about this time, it was my privilege to provide leadership to the first Idaho Conference, Seventh-day Adventist Women's Ministries Committee. "Yes, Lord, I'm still blooming where I am planted," I thought. "But sometimes, Lord, women do seem like 'the least of them, my brethren' so I will be a servant-leader right where you have placed me."

Does God Give Double Messages, or How's My Hearing?

Scanning the Idaho Statesman, our Boise newspaper, one evening, I came upon the "Personals" column. And I scanned down the usual litany of lonely hearts, thinking "What a desperate way to go looking for love and companionship!" when my eye caught one that was different. Hmmmm, it went like this:

57-year old (but younger than that) Caucasian man, Christian, non-smoker, non-drinker would like friendship with woman who enjoys the out-of-doors, photography, fly-fishing, dogs and horses. Mailbox (___).

I said to myself, "Bee, what is the worst thing that could happen if you were to answer this without divulging your address just as he did not?" And the answer seemed to be, "Do it!" A cheery, similar note to the personal ad, was posted the next day, but it was weeks before I received a response. In that first telephone conversation, this man named Ken and I found that we indeed had much in common, some mutual acquaintances, children about the same ages and a very real love for the Lord. Ken was a member of my favorite Methodist Church, a cathedral where I often attended services to be especially inspired by the great musical programs there.

Ultimately, we agreed to meet for a cup of tea. That cup of tea took four hours and ended with dinner! We enjoyed discovering that we eat similarly -- largely vegetarian --,we exercise, stay current with community and world events, nurture our spiritual selves, and both of us drive a pickup truck! So, we made a date for dinner for a week later.

Malawi Calls

It was December 10, 1989 when I was preparing to convene the first meeting of the new committee for Women's Ministries. I was also preparing for that first dinner date with Ken that evening. A telephone call changed the way I looked at everything!

It was Roger, an Idaho man married to a young woman I had known for years, calling me from Blantyre, Malawi, in Southeastern Africa. Roger was then the Malawi Director for the Adventist Development and Relief Agency (ADRA). He told me of a special project for the poorest of the poor children in Malawi who were dying unnecessarily of malnutrition, diarrhea, and vaccine-preventable diseases. The project would be funded seventy-five per cent by the United States Agency for International Development (USAID) and twenty-five per cent by ADRA. It would last for at least three years. He needed a qualified health professional to commit to planning, implementing, and operating the project until a native health professional could be found and trained to take over.

As Roger talked, it seemed there was a great video screen on fast-forward in my mind. I saw myself praying for God's direction as to how and where he wanted me to serve. I heard again, His assurances; I thought of my commitment to go anywhere He wanted me to go. I saw the completed "volunteer" form that I had left at my church's world headquarters. It was as though I could see neon like writing in my mind. It said, "This is God's answer, these are the least of these. Malawi is the uttermost part of the earth, and God wants you there, and He wants you there single -- not married to anyone." It only took a couple of minutes' discussion with Roger for me to say, "Yes, I will come." He said, "If you come as a volunteer, how long could you stay?" Knowing from experience that to change a community's health behaviors in the United States takes an intensively long time, I figured it must take twice as long in a primitive African culture, so I said, "I could stay two years." Roger expressed surprise and pleasure, for he said that most volunteers only commit to six weeks or three months at the most, and he thought that in just a few weeks we could have the project well under way.

As I closed that telephone call, I promised to send my resume to Roger and to FAX a copy to the Washington, DC headquarters for ADRA immediately, so that USAID could be notified of the fully qualified, volunteer Project Director for the ADRA Malawi Child Survival project. Roger told me that I would not leave for Africa for at least six months, so there would be time to convene my committee that morning, and to see Ken for dinner that night.

But oh, it was difficult to concentrate on leading the Women's Ministry Committee that morning! I knew that one of those members would need to fill the leadership chair in just a few months, but I dared not say a word that morning. Too many new thoughts were running through my head. But again, Jesus met my need and helped me to concentrate on our initial agenda that would ultimately set the pace to better serve Christian women and their families in Eastern Oregon and Southern Idaho.

CHAPTER 2

A Fine Romance For Me?

With just a brief break for freshening up after the committee meeting, I went to meet Ken for our first date. It was to be dinner that he prepared and then the movie, entitled "Dad" that my son Jay insisted I see. As Ken opened the door, he seemed just slightly nervous, talking a lot about inconsequential things at first. However, as he served up our dinner, I sensed a man who is comfortable in his own surroundings. His home was tastefully, but simply furnished, with a tropical fish aquarium gurgling in the living room, and every appointment as neat and "clean as a pin". As we enjoyed our meal and the conversation became a little more personal, Ken began to talk of all the plans that he had for us during that winter, the next spring, and summer. There would be skiing, exploring, dinners and musicals, and with the warmth of spring and summer, fishing and hiking! Even though it all sounded wonderful to me, I finally had to tell him that in a little while I would not be around, and that he should keep right on seeing some of those other "good ol' girls". He asked, "And where will you be going?" As I responded, "To Pennsylvania right after the holidays, and then, later in the year, to Africa", there was a dramatic silence while I watched his face change from animation to solemnity, from a healthy pink to a sort of ashen gray. His eyes fell, and his fingers began to toy with his napkin. I knew in that instant that this fine man with whom I had only begun an acquaintance on the telephone, was more than casually interested in me. Somehow, I felt protective of his feelings and felt that telling him the truth right up front would protect us both, since I was convinced that the Lord wanted me in Africa as a single woman. He seemed so eager to tell me of his past, of growing up in Colorado, of his years in the military, marriage to a Canadian, three beautiful daughters in their twenties and early thirties; of the years in alcoholism and his decision to get well, of treatment for the alcohol problem and success in being dry for over six years. He told me how he had quit smoking and chewing tobacco all at the same time as he relied on "his Higher Power" to give him the will to stick with the decision. He told me of a back injury and surgery; the broken jaw and its repair and even of some other chronic health conditions that sometimes take their toll of energies. I was surprised at his honesty and openness as he recounted most of his life story.

When he spoke of his joys (daughters and grandsons, fishing, the horses and dogs he once had) his blue eyes just danced. When he described his life as being "born and raised in Alamosa, Colorado, in the San Louis Valley," he seemed proud of that place. But his face lost expression as he told of a mother who seemed to have rejected him from birth; a mortician father who had little joy; stern grandparents with whom he spent as much time as possible, because they had a ranch, and horses and dogs!

He told a story of victory blunted by defeat when he had come out of alcoholism and back to his Methodist spiritual family, and his wife of thirty years would not join him.

Alcohol seemed to rule her life in many ways. Sober enough to carry out her work duties for a major corporation, she spent the evenings drinking, either at home or a neighborhood bar. He prayed for her healing, but the distance lengthened between them. He said that it is true, a former alcoholic who is sober cannot stand to be with people who are drinking; and an alcoholic cannot stand to be around people who are sober. Even though his wife had been seeing other men for many years Ken had tried to keep the appearance of an intact family and finish raising the three girls. He told me that he had been single for the past four years, and divorced for the past two.

I, too, was very frank with him, indicating how my grief was healing and that I had no unresolved baggage with my husband and lover of thirty-six years. Only the grief remained, which I said I knew would ultimately be softened and healed with time and loving relationships.

I had planned to spend the Christmas weekend with my son, Jay and his family, so I called Jay and asked him if I could bring my new friend with me for Christmas. Jay responded, “What is this guy’s name?” And I told him, “Ken Jarrell.” He chuckled and said, “Mom, ask him if he has a daughter named Debbie.” Ken said, “I surely do,” and Jay chuckled again and said, “If this is Debbie Jarrell’s dad, he must be all right! So, he is most welcome! Debbie and I worked together for several years at Bogus Basin Ski Resort. And she is one fine person!” And so, not seeming like a stranger to anyone, Ken joined some of my family in a snowy Christmas at Fairfield, Idaho.

However, Ken’s welcome was not universal! After Jay’s little girl, Shana and I had retired, we heard a knock on the bedroom door. It was Ken, looking distraught. It seems that Jay’s dog had curled up on Ken’s sleeping bag and was snarling at him to prevent him from getting in his own sleeping bag! We had to call Jay to remove his snarling Cocker Spaniel from Ken’s bed! Such a welcome!

A few days later I was off to my Pennsylvania visit, quite sure that, I would stay single. No matter that, this was a kind, clean, caring, Christian man who seemed to really appreciate me. I had almost begun to like my independent status as a widow. Making my decisions solo seemed so simple -- only the dog and the cat to consider, and they seldom complained.

As I left for Pennsylvania, I left several items with Ken. The first two were books, The Desire of Ages, a commentary on the life of Christ, by Ellen White, and the Seventh-Day Adventist book, 27 Beliefs. Besides my precious Bible, these books had helped form the basis for my love and devotion to Jesus and membership in the Seventh-day Adventist Church. Another item I left with him was my Pennsylvania phone number, and the fourth item was my pastor-son's phone number in Southern California where I intended to be for about three weeks. During my travels, I found I was talking to Ken nearly every day, and I really began to appreciate this thoughtful, kind person.

Ken was employed as a professional driver for a petroleum tanker and one day on the telephone, he asked what I had done with my dog, Sky, whom he had met just one time. I told him that she was in a boarding kennel not far from his house. He immediately asked if he could go get her because he knew she must be missing me. He said her companionship with him in the truck would be most welcome. I gave him my permission and phoned the kennel owners to let them know who would be picking up Sky ahead of schedule. In my mind, Ken's positive profile was expanding: he was thoughtful, caring, unselfish, sensitive, and kind.

In the meantime, in addition to the telephone chats, there came cards with precious thoughts on them. Then one day, there were a dozen red roses! My son began to be suspicious that there was something really between his mother and this stranger. So, when Ken would call, Bruce would intercept the call and kid this man he had never seen about so much attention being directed at his mother! We all enjoyed the three-way tease. Then one day, Ken called to say that there had been a major storm in the area and wondered if I would mind if he drove by my mountain home to see if everything was still all right. I thought, "This man continues to think of me, my home -- and my dog!" And I felt a lump of warmth in my throat, and an escalation in my regard for one who is so considerate of another's needs.

Ken called me to report that all was well at Clifcrest and that he had taken some photos of the January scene of the trees and stream below the house. He said that he had been reading those two books and could find nothing about which he could not agree. Then he added, almost casually, "You know, there really isn't any reason that I could not go to Africa with you!" I was speechless as I thought of several reasons why he could not go to Africa with me! The most important one being that I felt God had called me there as a single person, and that is what God intended. But I held Ken's suggestion in my heart, and began many conversations with Jesus about the pro's and con's of a deeper relationship with this dear man, asking God for even closer guidance.

As I prepared to return home to Clifcrest my son said, "Mom, what do you think is going to happen to you and this man, Ken?" I replied with a sudden flash of thought, but without hesitation, "Son, I will either marry him or break up with him right away, depending on God's direction." And Bruce responded, "Well, if it is marriage, may I do the honors of the wedding ceremony?" Again, a quick response for which I had never held a prior thought, "If I marry anyone again, I think it will be an elopement, because I just don't need a big wedding." And I was comfortable with this thought, even as Bruce was shaking his head in disbelief!

Returning to Idaho and home at Clifcrest, I found that the storm had done no damage and the wintry photos that

Ken had taken astounded me! It was not that I had not seen Clifcrest in winter dress, it was that the views he photographed were some of my favorite ones. But we had never stood there together. He had never heard me comment about the special beauty that surrounds my home. But, most amazing to me was that there was just one place that I could see from my house that I call my inspiration view. Ken had shot that with his camera. For years, since living there, I have stopped to drink in this special place. There is a riffle on the stream below, framed by a tall fir tree and an aspen that leans out over the water. This riffle never freezes over in the winter, and when I listen carefully, it sings a special song to me. That view that Ken had snapped had always spoken to me of vibrant life, of hope and of joy. And there it was in living color, captured by the man I was learning to love. I realized that we have a very deep, common appreciation for natural beauty. As I exclaimed over his seeing what I had especially enjoyed for years, he handed me that photo, enlarged and in a frame.

Then, as we stepped inside my home with its natural cedar finish, a comfortable fireplace, joyous Sky with her welcome wags, and that view of the canyon, Ken said, “We might not even go steady, but, would you please adopt me?” He felt like he had just come home.

When Ken asked me to marry him later that day, we knelt and asked God to give us special guidance for our decision. And I asked Ken for just twenty-four more hours to listen for direction from my heavenly Father who had been closer than my husband during the past four years. We eloped three weeks later!

It was sixteen degrees below zero (F.) that Valentine’s Day morning when we kept our appointment with my favorite judge, Patricia, in historic Idaho City. I remember driving into that little town in time to precede the set court docket. It was about seven, still quite dark and there was a frosty, full moon shining on us, causing the snowy banks of the road to sparkle in celebration of our wedding day! Ken pulled the Chevy pick-up to a stop just outside of town, and we bowed our heads and prayed again, asking God's blessing on this civil ceremony. We were full of joy and truly at peace with our decisions. I think that the glow we felt as we entered that one hundred-forty year-old Courthouse warmed the entire courtroom.

The Clerk of the Court and the Juvenile Probation Officer took their places to be our official witnesses, while a judicial client with a civil case for later in the day served as photographer using our cameras. Patricia's ceremony and instructions to the bride and groom were a beautiful litany of scriptural guidance and carefully thought out personal best wishes. We had informed my pastor of the planned elopement, but chose the civil ceremony because of its simplicity and that deep friendship with Patricia. Once Ken assured me of the depth of his spiritual commitment and we perceived no conflict in our religious values, we knew that God would bless this uniting of our hearts. We had not a single doubt.

That warm glow continued as we posted our announcements in beautiful downtown, historical, Idaho City, population 392, and as we spent the wintry day driving to North Yellowstone National Park and Mammoth Lodge. Winter in the geothermal, steaming park is idyllic with only a few people, gentler animals and nature's configurations of snow, hoarfrost, steam, and mineral design. We skied together out through the vent holes of rising steam and the bubbling mud pots. We visited the major beauty spots via snow-cat, returning to the lodge for meals. There were long evenings for listening to the Park Ranger, getting better acquainted with each other, and for talking of the adventure that lay ahead in Africa. It was like being on another planet with none of the trappings of everyday life to weight us down, just the pleasure of one another's company as the lodge staff pampered and cared for our needs.

Our drive back to Boise was in ferocious blizzard conditions. We stopped to pull another traveler out of a snow bank where his vehicle had skidded and stalled. A flat tire on our Chevie truck mandated that we drive off the freeway on an "on-ramp" to air up the tire enough to limp onto a tire store. Arriving back in Boise just in time to keep a training commitment with my pastor and several other couples, who will be learning "small group leadership." This was Ken's introduction to a few of the members of my church family, including my pastor. And how they welcomed him! The next day, as the seminar continued, the pastor ate lunch with us, and just because he cared so much for our success, spent time plying us with those "compatibility questions" that are ordinarily part of his pre-marital counseling! We both cared very much that he cared.

The next weekend we attended the Adventist church on Sabbath and the Methodist Cathedral of the Rockies on Sunday. Both were beautiful services and neither of us felt like strangers at the other's home church.

A Real Bed-burner Relationship!

The third Sunday of our marriage, we were preparing to drive the twenty-four miles to the Cathedral when we smelled smoke in our house on the mountain. Following the smell, we found our bed in flames! The fire extinguisher I had always kept in that upstairs bedroom refused to function. Ken ran for one from the garage that he knew would work, while I grabbed a water pot and threw water on the flames. The acrid, black smoke was beginning to have its effect as I could scarcely breathe. Ken returned with a large, powerful chemical extinguisher with which we were able to reduce the flames, and then we decided to carry the bed and bedding down the stairs and out the front door into the snow bank. As we ran back for the flaming box springs, Ken had to shoot them again with the extinguisher and also the carpet under the box, as flames leaped toward the ceiling. We made one more super-human trip down the stairs with the charred and flaming bed-frame dripping burning debris onto the stairway carpeting. Each time we re-entered the burning area we held our breaths until we were outside with our flaming burdens. Finally, we could throw open all the upstairs windows to let the black acrid smoke and soot out as much as possible.

The cause of the fire seemed to be a very old mattress heater that I had been given by an elderly lady when she learned that I was not sleeping much as a new widow. I had forgotten about it and the old cord had become broken, shorting out and starting the fire. Even as we assessed the cause and the significant damage to the floor and furnishings, we began to rejoice at how good God is. Had the fire started five minutes later, Ken and I would have been gone to church and our cedar home would have been a pile of ashes when we would have returned. God loved us so much that he took care of the timing of the fire, not preventing it, for we had several lessons to learn, but enabling us to be there and to put it out before all was lost.

We fell down on our knees in our sooty, soiled Sunday-go-to-meeting clothes and thanked God for enabling us to save our home. Then, we changed clothes in order to go to town and move the rest of Ken's tools and equipment from his little house, which was now already rented. When we returned some four hours later, the charred bed and bedding were laying outside on the snow bank. Soot and chemical fire retardant lay heavily over all the furniture inside; but there was something else! There on the dining table was a beautiful blooming plant, a cake, some packages and evidence that someone had been in our smoky house!

Just then, our next-door neighbors and three other couples showed up, having waited until we returned. So, we all just sat right down in the ashes mess and had a newly wed party! Our dear octogenarian neighbor wryly grinned and said, "You two sure must have been having a hot time this morning!" Of course, the burning bed story has entertained many. The Arthritis Aquatics class members whom I taught at the Boise YMCA even gave us a "bed-burning party" with a specially decorated cake in the shape and colors of a burning bed!

Some of our children were not too happy to be excluded from our marriage ceremony. They seemed to feel "left out" that we had eloped. We were not very surprised at this, but we felt right in keeping our special moment very private. Although I had the privilege of meeting all of Ken's daughters, their husbands and children, Ken had only met my eldest son, Jay in person. He had visited with the rest of my children on the telephone, but the only person we told that we would be marrying was my pastor, and he had kept our secret. It was not long until they all forgave us and began to accept our marriage as an unalterable (bad pun) fact!

Surgical Summer

Years of heavy work and advancing psoriatic arthritis, a type that is especially damaging to bones and joints, found Ken with both wrists very weak and painful. X-ray clearly showed the destruction of the wrist joint bones and he needed a surgical fusion with steel plates to stop the destruction and strengthen his hands. Having a special friend who was a hand surgeon in Denver, and being not too sure of the skills available in Boise, we made arrangements for the hand surgeries to be done at two different times. Just as the operating room was ready for Ken that June day in Denver, the clouds darkened the sky, the wind began to howl, and hailstones the size of grapefruit began to pelt the city. Windows were knocked out of the north side of the hospital, trees came crashing down, electrical power was off, and all we could do was wait inside the hospital. But as the theatre people say, "The show must go on," so Ken was soon taken to surgery. As soon as the storm blew past, I felt free to go out onto the parking lot to inspect our vehicle.

On the way to our little French-vanilla-ice-cream-yellow Nissan pick-up truck, I was appalled to see windshields shattered, head lights knocked out, glass everywhere from buildings and automobiles, and huge dents in all the surfaces of the several hundred vehicles in the hospital parking lot. Some people, also inspecting their cars, just stood there and wept. The Nissan truck was as bad a mess as all the rest, but enough of the windshield was intact so that it was drivable. I scraped the shattered glass off the seats and when Ken was out of recovery and being cared for by capable nurses, I drove to our friends' home where I was staying. About ten square miles of the city had been severely damaged. One elderly life was lost as the man was walking on the street; children were terrified as they were stranded in the ferris wheel at the nearby amusement park. The radio was urging everyone to find materials to cover their broken windows and to be patient with their insurance companies.

The next morning I contacted our insurance company and the auto glass people to learn that it would require two weeks to settle all the claims and have all the appropriate windshields in stock to meet the needs. However, the glass company with whom I dealt found that they had just one windshield to fit the Nissan and since we were from out of town and needing to leave for home that day, they made the repair. Our headlights were intact, but the cab and hood were really beaten up. However, we were able to make Ken comfortable with an overhead sling for his ice-wrapped wrist and had safe travel all the way home. The body and fender man in Boise was happy to have our job and soon that little truck looked as good as new.

The post-operative check-ups and second wrist surgery

kept us traveling between Denver and Boise quite a bit. In between surgeries, we were earnestly preparing for Africa.

When we decided to marry, I had called Roger in Malawi to tell him that I would be bringing a fine new husband with me and asked, "What do you think of that?" Roger seemed delighted, assuring me that there was much practical work to be done, and that Ken and his skills would be very welcome.

As we shared the mission to Malawi plans with friends, they often showed cynical amazement, often asking, "What good can a couple of elderly people do amid all the poverty, disease, ignorance, and death there?" "Aren't you afraid of catching AIDS?" We responded that we felt a special calling to Africa and that we did not expect to do anything spectacular, but that if we could make life better for one or two of "the least of these" we knew that we will have done it for Jesus. Nobody we knew encouraged us to go. But each time we received another packet from Malawi, or from the ADRA International offices, we became even more excited and sure that there was much that we could attempt, in Jesus' name.

One friend asked what we would do with our houses, Clifcrest, and Ken's house that was now a rental. We simply said that they would be in the hands of a property management company, and we felt sure that Jesus would find the right people to occupy both of them while we would be gone. "But your home will never be the same again after someone else lives there!" Our response was, "So what if the home will not be the same -- we will not be the same, either."

In between the casts on Ken's arms (one at a time) and the cast covers and the trips to and from Denver, there were passports to obtain, photos to be made and sent, immunizations to acquire and even preventive medicine to take to ward off the Malaria that is prevalent all of the time in southern Malawi. We obtained books on sub-Sahara

Africa, maps and all of the information we could find that would teach us and prepare us for this chosen destination. We thought about studying Swahili language, but Roger laughed as we talked on the phone, "Wrong language -- it is Chichewa here, and quite easy to learn."

Perhaps the best learning came from a little book that we heard had been banned by the Malawi government. Entitled, Africa on a Shoestring , by Geoff Crowther, this book described tiny Malawi as half the land mass of Idaho, with about ten million people, (Idaho's population then was one million). Crowther described Malawi's President-for-Life as a dictator, indicating that his research showed that President Banda had created a very corrupt government, with all major businesses and land owned by the elite government ministers, and that Banda, himself owned all but one share of the 5,000 shares of Press Holdings, a conglomerate of companies with wide interests that included an agricultural subsidiary. This accounts for an estimated 30% of the country's economic activity."

We learned of Malawi's climate, mostly hot: hot and dry or hot and wet!; crops of maize, rice, cotton, sugar cane, peanuts, guar beans, rubber, macadamia and cashew nuts, tea, coffee, tropical fruits and fish. It took 100 tambala to equal one qwacha and it took fourteen qwacha to equal one US dollar. Except for one major north-south Highway, Malawi's roads are not much more than an ox-cart trail or foot path; however, Malawi Airlines services Mzuzu in the North, Lilongwe, the capitol city and Blantyre, the southern commercial hub city. Busses run regularly to main cities and large bomas (villages). Twenty percent of Malawi is under water in the beautiful "lake of stars," Lake Malawi. Nostalgic steamer ships service lakeshore villages and some resorts. National Parks in all regions of the nation are home to lions, leopards, elephants, water buffalo, and over a dozen types of antelopes, exotic birds, besides many reptiles and small animals. The book warned of a fifteen-year civil war in adjoining Mozambique in these terms, "Even if you are given permission by the authorities to attempt a visit to Mozambique, there's a very good chance you'll either be shot or taken hostage. Forget it!"

We were entranced with a land we had never seen. Ancient, but modern; civilized, but not quite; beautiful, but degraded and polluted; primitive, but contemporary in so many ways. Thousands of children are dying for the sheer ignorance of their parents. Thousands of parents are dying from AIDS and AIDS-related diseases. Surely, we could help teach a few of the "least of these" a better way.

We continued to learn all we could about our destination. My son, Jay applied a new cover to the forbidden book, "Africa on a Shoestring," and wrote a new cover title, "Trout Fishing in America," so it would be less apt to be confiscated by customs authorities, should they come across it!

One day, after a special "Holy Spirit-focused" retreat with a few friends and our Pastor at Camp Ida Haven, Ken pulled up a chair closely, facing mine and said, "Honey, we don't need to continue to attend two churches. Your church family has so warmly accepted me, and I have never before felt such love from any church, that I just want to concentrate my spiritual home in this one place -- with you, at the Boise Cloverdale Seventh-day Adventist Church." In my heart, I was delighted, even though I thoroughly enjoyed attending his Cathedral. Therefore, I responded, "That is O.K. with me, but please promise me that we can attend the Cathedral at least every Easter and at Christmas time because their music ministry is so outstanding!" Then, one Sabbath evening we were considering some scripture thoughts when Ken suddenly said, "Oh, yes... I want to be baptized. I have never been baptized!" Silently, I thanked Jesus for this voluntary commitment to be totally God's person. I smiled and said, "Whenever you are ready for baptism, just telephone to pastor Don Driver, and he will make the arrangements." Changing religious persuasions may seem quite simple, but I know that kind of change is a deepest heart matter. Knowing myself to be strong-willed, I did not want anyone to say that I had somehow forced Ken to accept my belief system. On Ken's call to the pastor, they spent a few hours praying and searching the scriptures together, with Ken confirming his belief and committing his life to the Lord. So one warm Sabbath afternoon, after the first wrist surgery, Ken wore a bright yellow cast protector and walked into the Boise River at a quiet place with Pastor Driver. About fifty friends gathered on the banks of that river to sing, praise, and pray for Ken's unity with God and a more complete unity with me, his bride.

Ready, Set, Go!

Acquiring necessary equipment and arranging shipment took the better part of two months. Roger suggested that we bring our own computer and printer, a queen-size bed, bedroom-size air conditioner and a clothes washer and drier. He assured us that we would easily sell all of this equipment whenever we returned to the US. We also included a few clinical books, a few pots, pans and dishes, and a few cozy things and family pictures to make us feel at home in whatever kind of lodging we might have.

A pastoral family from Boise asked if they might be the ones to live at Clifcrest and care for the dog and cat. After checking one another out and describing the responsibilities that go with a home in the mountains where the snows often pile deeply, we agreed that this was the family. We felt that they must have been sent by God. We engaged a small property management company in case of changes in occupants of either house and/or the need to arrange for repairs.

En route to Malawi, we spent one week in Washington, DC, being oriented to third world development theory, existing Child Survival work in Nepal and Nicaragua and the expectations of ADRA International and the United States Agency for International Development (USAID). Some overseas ADRA employees and volunteers were present and it was here that Ken was to meet Roger, who came from Malawi to begin initial planning work with us.

Two days before we were to enplane, we received word from the Boise property manager that the couple in our home had already moved elsewhere, due to the mental illness of the wife/mother. This threw us onto the expertise of the property managers and their choice of someone to live in our fully furnished home and care for our dog, Sky. At this point, we asked my son, Jay to take our old cat to his home in Twin Falls and care for her. Within a few days, a lovely couple from Florida found our house for lease. They bonded with Sky at once and fully enjoyed Clifcrest in our absence. You see, God knew and guided just the right people to meet our need and appreciate Clifcrest.

Flying from Dulles International Airport in Washington, via London and Amsterdam, we arrived in Malawi, “The Warm Heart of Africa” on the American Thanksgiving Day, November 1990. We were both very tired from the long trip; however, I had slept on the plane while Ken had not. Instead, he observed the flaming sunrise over the Sahara, and saw a stunning view of Mt. Kilimanjaro in southern Kenya under the plane’s wing tip.

CHAPTER 3

First Impressions

We were met at Blantyre's Chileka Airport by the American officials for the Adventist Church in Malawi, who expressed great joy at our arrival to be part of the development of this needy nation through ADRA-Malawi. We remember it was just about sunset as we left the airport, driving through villages of mud, bamboo, and thatch with the evening flare of outside cooking fires. We came into the modern city of tall, upscale buildings, double-decker buses, plenty of automobiles and lorries all driving on the "wrong side of the road," crowds of people walking, and awesome smells. Such sensory contrasts in just those few minutes.

Our quarters consisted of a one-room guest cottage with bath and a modern kitchenette. We were very grateful to be able to shower and stretch out; took a few minutes to freshen up and then walked to the nearby church hall where potluck Thanksgiving dinner was under way, for, and by all the Adventist Americans working within the nation. There were physicians, nurses and technicians from the one-hundred years old Malamulo Hospital; the Dentist and

Optometrist and their families from the capitol city of Lilongwe; the pastor of the Kabula Hill S.D.A church and his family; and of course, the full clinical staff of Americans at Blantyre Adventist Hospital. What a party was going on! Even the American style foods seemed different, and I realized they were different because of unavailability of some of the customary ingredients. It seems that Swiss people enjoy American holidays. Swiss Dr. Peter and his wife Vrenni Jaggi served as our hosts, introducing us to approximately fifty people. Then I missed Ken and someone called me outside. There he was, miserably bent over and very sick to his stomach. The long flight, lack of sleep, excitement and some strange foods were just too much. Somehow, we managed to get him home to that little cottage near the home of the Chief of Medical Staff on the hospital grounds. We both slept for about twelve hours.

These beautiful hospital grounds with their blooming trees and shrubs were the headquarters for Blantyre Adventist hospital, the ambulatory Clinic facility, at least a dozen residences and for the Adventist Church in Malawi. The ADRA office adjoined the church offices and I was shown to my desk and a computer and introduced to the church employees with whom we became great friends. Modern Blantyre services included telephones that worked and reached across the nation or around the world, electrical power, a public sewer system with indoor toilets that flushed, and somewhat reliable running water that needed to be boiled for drinking purposes. Most of the time these things worked, and at least once a week there was a breakdown in the water system. We were pleasantly surprised with these modern conveniences and learned to be patient with the less than perfect water system. Bougainvillea in many colors bloomed everywhere. The flame trees were in full bloom along with fragrant frangipani. A little later lavender hued jacaranda trees lined the driveways here and across the town.

In my severe jet-lag, I slept nearly around the clock the next day while Ken strolled around to get the lay of the land. The second morning I was invited by the ADRA Director to a welcoming breakfast at the Sochi Hotel, a lovely place just a block from the office. He told me I would meet some important allies in our Child Survival project. In addition, indeed, two men joined us. I do not remember the breakfast particularly, but I met the Malawian Pastor/Director for all Seventh-day Adventist efforts in the nation. His title was "Director, Southeast Africa Union, Seventh-day Adventists." I asked why his title was not "President" since world- wide, his counterparts in similar positions are called "President," but he informed me that in Malawi there is just one President and that is the President-for-Life, His Excellency the Kamuzu Hastings E. Banda. This was my first lesson in a totalitarian nation. The other person joining us for breakfast was Paul Courtright, Ph.D., Director of the International Eye Foundation in Malawi. Paul is an Epidemiologist, very personable and was operating many eye services throughout Malawi. Nevertheless, the exciting news to me was that his home had been in Boise, Idaho, and we had many mutual friends! We agreed to meet again soon for some partnership work in Child Survival.

Within a week, we were pleasantly surprised again, to find that we could move from the one-room cottage to a three-room modern flat, upstairs over the clinic. One of the Americans said that she would have the "bambos" come help us move our luggage and boxes. "Bambos" –"What is a bambo?" I wondered. Ken said he did not know. I wondered if it might even be a disrespectful term, so was careful not to say, "Hi, Bambo" to these bright, smiling, energetic men who emerged and swiftly moved all our gear up the stairs into our entry, without letting us lift a finger to help. Besides knowing how to move our stuff, these bambos knew how to stand, almost at attention, to wait for that tip of a few tambalas. A soon as I saw another American, I asked, “Tell me, -- what does the word ‘Bambo’ mean?” She explained that it is a most respectful term for an adult male and actually means, “Daddy” in Chichewa. I was very relieved with my first lesson in this foreign language.

From the large balcony of our flat, we had a view of the city and the fragrances of the Chinese restaurant just next door and below us. We did not always call those odors “fragrances,” but they were nearly always present, especially on the warmest days. I asked Ken, “What are all these bones lined up on the balcony railing, parched white by the sun?” We wondered if they were some sort of voodoo practiced by some former inhabitant. So we left those bones right there. The next morning we were raucously awakened at dawn by the screeching and cawing of crows on the balcony. These were not ordinary crows, they wore tuxedos! They had all shiny black feathers except their chests were white, and they were twice as large as Idaho crows. What a welcoming committee they presented! Those white parched bones were their toys! They had brought them up from the garbage pile behind the Chinese restaurant and picked them clean on our balcony railing. This was the crows’ dining room!

It seemed that from the moment of our arrival, even with the weariness of jet travel halfway around the world, our senses were attuned acutely to the strange smells, sights, and sounds of Malawi. Along with the habits of the crows, we were awakened and alerted five times each day with the haunting, loudspeaker assisted, Muslim call to prayer. Only two blocks away was a mosque with its walls and minarets and the public speaker that carried the chanting wail of the call to prayer.

We soon learned of the deep Muslim influence into the Malawi culture and economy. The major dealers in hardware, dry goods, plastics, and manufactured items were Asian merchant people. Hence, the major employers (other than the government) were the Asian merchants. Most of these merchants were second and third generation Malawi citizens whose forebears had migrated from India. Word travels fast among this Asian community, for soon we were greeted by them with a smile as "the ADRA people."

Less than two blocks away, the Soche and Ryals hotels contributed to the after-dark sounds with live modern rock music interspersed with the repetitive songs and chants of the African pop scene. At first, it was difficult to get to sleep with competing sounds wafting into our open windows. For a while, we used foam earplugs to diminish the sound, because the windows caught the evening breezes and it was essential to keep them open. Only a few weeks passed before we could sleep peacefully through the night sounds! Modern in every respect, we appreciated these hotels for an occasional fine meal or a peaceful break in their coffee shops.

Everywhere people were walking, walking, and walking. Often with large burdens on their heads, they hurried, barefooted, to their destinations. Many carried bundles of firewood that might have been purchased under the trees in the market or, otherwise, gathered from along the stream banks and sparse forests just outside of town. Others were carrying goods to sell at the market: either produce they had grown (squash, cooking greens, or beans), a live chicken, or basketry or carvings they had made.

On every street corner and often in between, there sat the beggars. Some were old and blind; some were skinny, crippled children; many were sickly and could scarcely hold out their begging hand. Our hearts were wrenched many times a day. I learned to pray and ask God to show me which beggar to help today, with my few tambalas. There were so many, and all seemed pathetically needy. Usually, my attention rested by Holy Spirit guidance on a blind grandmother or the very ill appearing person.

As modern as the city of Blantyre seems, it is here the ancient and modern customs meet and often clash. With the encroaching modern and mostly Western culture. It is a city of paradoxes. The very clean ambience of the three banks and the supermarket contrast with the squalor and filth of street vendors under trees hawking everything imaginable. I was often fascinated to see impeccably dressed business people, both men and women, walking out to lunch at a sidewalk cafe, and literally stumbling over a very filthy beggar with flies buzzing all about him. Such stark contrast.

At dusk on that first Saturday evening, Ken and I decided to take a long walk. The scent of smoke was heavy, almost acrid, in the air and the sun had disappeared as a red ball behind a dark curtain of smoke. We walked to the edge of Kabula Hill, where the tarmac paving ends and the steep descent begins leading through the banana trees to the outskirts of Blantyre and the sprawl of thousands of thatch, mud, and bamboo huts. Stopping there under the fading purple jacaranda trees, we saw for the first time, close up and stretching almost as far as we could see, the flickering flames of the small cooking fires just outside each hut. The smoke of the fires ascended and accounted for part of that heavy mantle of smoke over the city. As we took in this sight of the sprawling valley below us, the sound of drumming and singing began, first from a near village, then joined by another song and another drummer from a far away village. Goose bumps played on my bare arms, appropriately treated with repellent for the mosquitoes, as I began to assimilate the texture of the scene and listened and smelled the fragrance of those nearby fires and the foodstuffs steaming in thousands of pots.

As night fell, we stood there entranced, but something attracted our attention far beyond the villages. It was as though the sky was on fire just at the horizon. We could just barely see that the flames were actually from the hills that swept upward on that horizon and the fires were burning dry, agricultural fields and wild brush. This then seemed to further account for the heavy, stinging mantle of smoke that had settled over the November evening. Still enchanted by the fires in the foreground and concerned about the fires framing the horizon, we were awed as the great circle of light from the moon began to rise over those burning hills.

Long tendrils of smoke rose between the earth and that moon, causing the lunar outline to be indistinct, fuzzy, changing in shape, and the light from the moon to lose its clarity and intensity. In this smoky moment, my mind drew a parallel from the seemingly smoking moon. Is this why we are here? To sweep the smoke away from the light of knowledge? To clear the air of old cultural behaviors that spelled death and disease? To somehow help to cleanse the atmosphere of ignorance and doubt? To shine a clear light on a better way to live so that children need not die before they could live? Could it be possible that the moon smoke was a metaphor of the needs of the people of the Nsanje bush whom we had not yet even seen but with whom we were soon to become intimately acquainted? This smoky, flickering view seemed to be a visual metaphor of our calling in this natural primitive world of fire, pollution, and destruction. We can never forget it, the Malawi moon smoke symbol for our challenge to go, teach, cleanse, clear, enlighten, encourage, and to serve with the help of our God.

We finally turned to walk back to the tarmac toward the one dim streetlight between the hospital grounds and us. People were scurrying quickly toward the street light, crouching, and making quick "picking" movements with their hands, happily shouting to each other. "What is this?" we asked each other. We were unnoticed as we walked quietly closer to see these people -- men, women, and children -- catching flying insects and popping some in their mouths and some into paper or plastic bags they carried. We wondered, "What are they catching and eating?" So that we would not embarrass them or ourselves, by asking. we just went on walking when a well-dressed man, who spoke English had stopped his own quest to explain. "This is the night that the white ants hatch; they are drawn to the light and, in the few moments of their life cycle that they have to fly, their wings drop off and they fall to the ground. They are a Malawian's delicacy, have a wonderful nutty-sweet flavor, but I like mine the best when we quick-fry them and add a little salt!" He was completely at ease telling us about this delight, and we thanked him as we tried to hide our astonishment, and hurried on home to our mosquito-protected flat as those critters began buzzing about our heads. We were simply incredulous about this awesome evening.

Malawi - Up Close and Personal

Conducting any business, understanding the government, and meeting the people we were to serve, -- required all new ways of relating. Blantyre banks operated much like the banks of England, for after all this country was only twenty-five years away from having been a British colony. I remembered that when I studied world geography in elementary school, Malawi was called Nyassaland and was ruled by the British. It took about an hour and a-half just to open a commercial checking account, standing in lines of up to a hundred people, getting all documents reviewed, then reviewed again and approved. At the conclusion of the approval process, the higher authority placed his hand-held rubber stamp on the document with a resounding BANG! Moreover, wherever we went for official government permits or approvals, there was the importance of the official rubber stamp, with a BANG! It seemed that there could be no real show of authority without that loud thump! The official clerk would look up with a smile of satisfaction and his personal approval as he handed us the necessary papers. (We say "his" particularly because there are very few women in business in Malawi. This is beginning to change -- more about that later.)

To withdraw or deposit funds required queuing up again and again for a double and triple check of all documents, including our passports, and another hour and a-half. I used this time to watch the people, listen to their interactions, some speaking in English, others in Chichewa or Portuguese, and watching the panoply of human relationships.

When old friends meet in Malawi, there is a very vigorous handshake often beginning with a wide swing as hands approached hands and then a "pop" as palms meet, then the changing positions of the hands, shaking again in about three positions. If the greeters were two men, they could be seen then walking away holding hands and swinging along, talking animatedly. The outstanding feature of women's handshakes was the wide swing and the "pop" sound. However, women seldom hold hands with one another as men do. They never hold hands with their husband in public; and they never share even a goodbye kiss with their husbands in public.

The government of the nation was upon the shoulders of the President for Life, His Excellency Hastings E. "Kamuzu" Banda, and his single party Parliament. Although the incumbent leadership claimed Malawi to be a single-party democracy, there was no freedom of the press or radio. There were no television stations, and most of the manufacturing, commercial businesses were owned by the very elite few, with the President owning the controlling interest in most businesses. Personal freedoms could be limited at the edict of His Excellency. One could not photograph any government building or institution, including schools, banks, bridges, and even hospitals, without being investigated. Police and military inspections and roadblocks were at the whim of the local law enforcement officials, however, police could not carry guns. Private citizens could not own or carry guns. Women were not allowed to wear pants or shorts, the principle being that women must look like women and at least have the knees covered at all times. Never mind that it was perfectly all right for women to go topless as the weather and/or activity moved them to do!

Primary schools were well distributed throughout the nation, recently helped along by donor nations and organizations such as World Vision. However, there was a school fee, and uniforms were required, so that the poorest of the poor children did not go to school. Secondary schools were not so well dispersed in the communities, and fees were higher, although uniforms were not required. Colleges were still scarcer with the University of Malawi (UM) located in the former colonial capitol city of Zomba. There were extensions of UM in the new capitol city of Lilongwe and in Blantyre as well as the Malawi Polytechnic College in Blantyre. Therefore, for learning there was a hierarchical selection process beginning with primary school where boys were the highest priority. Only those girl children could attend whose parents could afford the fees and replace the "lost labor" in the village of the girl in school, by paying someone else's daughter to carry the water and hoe the fields, and tend the smaller children.

For secondary school, the favored attendees included mainly young people whose parents were fully employed in government at the higher level. Several secondary boarding schools existed to accommodate students whose homes were too far distant and, again, whose parents were in that small minority of five-to-ten percent of the population who held good paying jobs. Many of the secondary students were in their twenties and thirties because they had worked to earn enough to afford secondary school, and they knew that with that preparation they could find better paying jobs.

Therefore, as for college, only the brightest and most

wealthy families could afford that level of education. Very few young women attended college. A closer look at Malawi education by certain of the United Nations donors' group at that time resulted in harsh criticism of the Malawi Ministry of Education for failure to provide incentives to educate girls and to demonstrate a fifty percent equal gender balance in those demonstration schools that received development funding from donor nations.

As strangers to the people and their culture, Ken and I had read everything that we could find to study the demography, ecology, and culture of the nation as well as that of the Nsanje District in the southernmost tip. Because the President-for-Life had obtained a medical degree (MD) degree in the United States and was ordained as an elder in the Presbyterian Church in the sister city of Blantyre, Scotland, he cherished both his education and his religion. Therefore, he had personally designed the good educational system. In addition, he had proclaimed that Bible Knowledge and English Language would be taught in all twelve grades from Primary, Standard 1, to Secondary, Form 4. He proclaimed Malawi as a Christian nation, but he outlawed certain religious groups, e.g. the B'Hai and Jehovah's Witnesses. His government had been particularly hard on Asian citizens in recent years. In an effort to strengthen the black Malawian rule, Asians of East Indian descent, were ordered out of the rural towns and forced to relocate mainly in Blantyre, where the government could keep a closer watch over their merchandising and manufacturing profits. Most of the Asian-occupied buildings in Blantyre were marked with a giant red star to indicate that the building would be torn down soon by the government to make way for modernization. This "notice" to Asians tended to keep them on guard and a trifle uneasy. Because of fears of government take-over of their businesses, most Asians transported their money to banks out of the country in the United Kingdom or elsewhere.

Many Asians had dual citizenship in other countries should they have to flee at some time. However, it was our experience that most of the obviously profitable businesses were owned by Asians and that the Malawian entrepreneurs were not yet ready, philosophically or educationally, to compete in a free, non-subsidized market economy. However, the black Malawian is bright, energetic, hard working, and ever longing to move fully into a free society. We observed that black Malawians at that time still needed the support of their Asian neighbors; they needed to learn from them through being employed by them; and they needed, from time to time, to step out on their own. This was beginning to happen. It seemed a strange, hate-love relationship between the largely Christian, black Malawi community and the mainly Muslim, Asian Malawians. We often felt that tension as we dealt with both aspects of the society.

Getting to Know Them With Mr. Welton Singano

Our objectives for the first three months of our stay were to get acquainted with the Regional and District officials of the Malawi Ministry of Health. This was to establish an advisory committee; to be oriented to the target area, some seventy to one-hundred and fifty kilometers distant from Blantyre where we stayed temporarily. We wrote the Detailed Implementation Plan (DIP) for Child Survival, as required by USAID. Between the day of our arrival in late November and January 15 of the new year 1991, most government offices were closed due to Christmas and New Year's celebrations and the after effects of that "celebration"! This gave us all the time we needed to spend several days just becoming oriented to "the lay of the land" as we rented a Toyota Hi-Lux pick-up with its camper shell to travel from 70 to 150 kilometers down into the fertile and very hot Lower Shire Valley where the project was to be.

Split by the mighty Shire River, the valley villages were mostly clustered here and there, closely along the banks of the river. We soon learned locations and the social profiles of the East Bank villages and the West Bank villages. It was fascinating to observe young men in their dug-out canoes made from tree trunks, casting their nets for fish, building fish-traps along the shore, and hauling their catch back for drying in the sun, or for smoking and to be sold in the village markets. Women and children tilled the fields with hand hoes, herded the scrawny cattle, and tended family life and marketing/bartering in the villages.

Wherever we went, we were items of curiosity to young and old alike. Nevertheless, it was the children who charmed us, shouting out "Hey, Zungu!" The deeper into the valley we traveled, the more pathetic the children were. They exhibited poverty, malnutrition, and disease even to the untrained eye. Most children wore no clothes at all, and their bloated parasite-laden bellies and skinny arms and legs told the story of poor hygiene, and malnutrition. Many of the boys wore plastic market bags with the bottom corners cut out so they could pull them on like pants and tie them around their waist. Most of the girls were naked until we appeared, when they would wrap an old, dirty rag around them like a sarong. Adult women were usually hoeing in their gardens, sometimes far from their mud, bamboo and grass-thatch huts. Many had a ragged cloth (we soon learned to call a "chitenji") hanging down from their waists to below the knees, while they were bare from the waist up. Often I had to consciously remind myself not to stare as they bent from the waist, chopping and hoeing with their little dried up breasts beating in rhythm against their chests.

It was hot -- oh, so hot! In addition, it was the rainy season when an inch or two of wind-driven rain could fall in one shower. Then the sun could come out, so that we always felt a bit wet, either from the splash of warm rain, or the drip of perspiration. During one of these rainstorms, we were impressed with the hard-working drive these wonderful people have. As the pelting rain scooped up new young maize plants and was washing them away, entire families would carefully pluck the plants away from the flood and mud, and then when the sun came out again, there they were, men, women, and children, resetting damaged maize plants into the wet earth. Some seasons the storms destroy the new crops of maize, cotton, guar beans, rice and red beans, and the people literally starve until the second planting can be harvested. In other seasons, no rain falls, and if the seeds can germinate, the young plants soon wither and die. The Shire Valley can grow three crops in the ideal year; but it can dry up and burn in many an off year.

We encountered many problems during these early explorations. It was necessary to carry along a jug of safe drinking water because most of the village water supplies were contaminated, and water had to be boiled for safety. It was also smart to pack a lunch because the only roadside restaurants we checked into were dingy. Plastic or tin dishes and utensils were often grimy and flies were everywhere. Now, toileting along the way was the most difficult puzzle. In all the villages we visited, we never did find a public latrine. It was not long until we learned that we were welcome to visit the Catholic Parish house, or the Trinity Hospital, or the personal latrine of one of the village leaders with whom we quickly became acquainted. We kept with us a good supply of foil-wrapped, moist towelettes for personal use.

Another problem was in saying "No" to the hundreds of people who asked for a ride. Often we had with us an interpreter, a pastor, or an ADRA dignitary, but it did not matter to the average Malawian on the street as long as he could see that a little room remained in the vehicle. He or she would try to wave us to a stop, and if we were stopped already, would plead for us to give him or her a lift to some place "not far." In the Malawian mind, the only way to use a vehicle efficiently is to load it, preferably with warm, black bodies, until the rear bumper drags the ground, and then remove one body, so you can drive away! With so few vehicles cruising those bush roads, it was difficult for us to hold to the full capacity of our vehicle, no matter what we were driving.

We also soon learned that there are two kinds of would-be passengers: those who expect to pay for their "lift," and those who would just like a ride, but have no kwacha with which to even think about paying. Those who expect to pay stand beside the road with a very big, toothy grin, waving one hand up and down in an effort to get the driver to stop. Catching a ride like this, and paying is called "traveling matola." Moreover, they all swear it is much faster and surer than riding the government's dirty, broken down, crowded buses.

Those who cannot pay, but would just like a "lift" often will get the local police officer to stop your vehicle, look inside, and ask what your destination is. That answered, the police officer may say, "This is my sister -- she needs to go to see her husband in the hospital. It is not far, but right on your way. You do have room for her." Unless the driver protests immediately, the police officer will open a door and help his "sister" in, along with two other women and three children! This happened to us several times, and interestingly, we found we enjoyed the experience.

Driving on the left side of the road was the least of our driving concerns. Just steering clear of the masses of people walking on the road required a very quick mind and good reflexes. In between the people would be a herd of cows, goats, or pigs, or chickens, or the strange rag-tag African sheep. Then there were the unpredictable bicycles, often with two people on them, and the occasional government worker on a motorcycle. None of these seemed to have any rules. The drivers of other four-wheeled motor vehicles, especially the buses, seemed to have very little sense of common courtesy. Defensive driving every moment behind the steering wheel saved our lives many times. Yet, when we would meet these same people on the street or in the market, they were always so kind, gentle, and courteous.

To break us into this new culture easily, the area we would serve and the community leaders there, Roger arranged for a Medical Assistant named Welton Singano to accompany us to the valley several times. These were long one-day trips, returning to the city of Blantyre and our little modern flat at night. Roger expected us to locate and arrange for office space in the only town in the Lower Shire Valley that has somewhat of a dependable community water supply and full time electricity. He also expected us to find housing somewhere in the valley. Mr. Singano was most helpful to us, introducing us to government officials, private hospital administrators, village chiefs and headmen and the staff of the Leprosy Clinic that was affiliated with the well-known, hundred year old, S.D.A. flagship, bush hospital, Malamulo.

Yes, I said Leprosy! Arriving when we did, leprosy had ceased to be a community health threat for Malawi people and most of this clinic's work focused on general primary care. The occasional case of leprosy among the Malawi people could be safely treated at home under the supervision of bicycling Talres Leprosy Clinic workers. However, the civil war in Mozambique was still raging, and refugees fleeing Mozambique were bringing uncontrolled, untreated leprosy with them. Therefore, this clinic had resumed full services for leprosy, as well as still offering its local primary care services. We were pleased to rent office space from this clinic and their staff turned out to be some of our best friends and co-workers.

Wherever we went with Mr. Singano, the people remembered him, since his home village was on the East Bank of the river and he had worked in the Leprosy program. He was a joyful man and always had a funny story to tell. One story we liked was about the Cow, the Dog, and the Goat. “Once upon a time,” he said, “the Cow, the Dog and the Goat were walking along the tarmac road when a man driving an empty lorry came by and yelled at them, ‘Hey Cow, hey Dog, hey Goat, – want a ride? If you do, jump in!’ Without hesitation, the three animals jumped into the back bed of the lorry and the driver took off, shouting over his shoulder ‘Just stomp your foot or bark whenever you want off.’ After a short distance, the Cow stomped her foot and the driver stopped while the Cow jumped down near a nice green field. Cow asked the driver ‘How much for the lift?’ and the driver said, Well, that was not far, how about five tambala?’ Therefore, the Cow paid the driver and swishing her tail at the flies, she ambled into the grass, thinking, ‘Well that was a nice thing to happen to me. After all, I gave my manger for the Christ-child and I owe no man a thing. I am just happy to pay my way and find this nice grassy field.’

“The driver gunned his motor and took off in a cloud of dust. Only a few kilometers the Goat stomped his foot and yelled, ‘Hey, driver, let me off!’ The lorry was just about to stop, when the Goat, with a mighty leap, took off through the thistles and thorn trees. Never for a moment did he look back, nor did he bother to ask the lorry driver what he owed him for the lift. Astonished and shaking his head, the lorry driver drove on with only the Dog left as a passenger. Suddenly, the Dog barked and yelped, demanding, ‘Let me off here!’ He politely went to the driver’s side of the cab and asked, ‘How much for my lift?’ The driver hesitated, and then said ‘That is fifty tambala’. The dog looked surprized, but said, ‘All I have is one kwacha, equal to 100 tambala.’ The lorry driver, holding out his hand, said ‘That’s all right, I’ll take it.’ Before Dog could ask, ‘Where’s my change?’ the lorry and the driver and the kwacha were gone in a cloud of dust with the Dog chasing after, barking excitedly, saying ‘Where’s my change? where’s my change?’ The driver shouted over the wind and dust, 'That's what Dog gets for running around with that cheating Goat. I have to have my money some way!"' "That is why, as we drive our automobiles up and down Malawi's few tarmac roads. we see the peaceful Cow, ambling ever so slowly across the road with her clear conscience. And we see the Goat running away from the road, with as much speed as she can muster, and we then knew she was guilty of cheating, and Dog, who is always barking at and chasing vehicles today, is still looking for his change!"

I will always be grateful to Mr. Singano, the Medical Assistant, who introduced us to that enormous valley, to the village and government leaders, and to the precious people whom we would serve. His introduction of the Child Survival Project and us to officials in the target villages probably was the single most valuable success factor, enabling our early acceptance as capable and knowledgeable health workers.

More… Up Close and Personal

My work objectives, set somewhat by USAID along with my agency, ADRA, were time-bound in order to plan the project, its scope and detailed activities and strategies for implementation. We would need to locate and set up a headquarters, somewhere near the target district. We needed to find housing for ourselves. We must establish an advisory committee to guide the planning, implementation and evaluation. We could then recruit, train and deploy volunteers to conduct a survey of the target villages about each family's health knowledge, attitudes, and practices. Then we could achieve the goal to recruit and begin nine weeks of training before deploying 24 mid-level village health workers. We set ourselves on achieving all but the nine-week training within the next three months.

Malawi's Ministry of Health had an existing category of workers, called Health Surveillance Assistants (HSAs) which we used as a basis for our expanded curriculum that ultimately would enable either the project HSAs to be fully employable by non-governmental organizations (NGOs) or the decentralized units of the Ministry of Health. One of the key features of ADRA's planning was for the long-range sustainability, usefulness, and continuity of what we were beginning. It is the hope that the program would be integrated with other similar NGOs and the governments' services so that the positive change our project would begin could be sustained by one mechanism or another.

Arriving just prior to the international holidays of Christmas and New Years Day, we used our time for orientation, and studying the demography, vital statistics, what few there were. At that time, Malawi had no national birth or death registry! We searched for data about the economy and politics of our Nsanje District and the nation. We found that from one week before Christmas, until the middle of January, either the Malawi government offices were closed, or they had a very small staff. When we asked the reason for such a near-shut-down, we were told that the main mode of celebration is drinking, and with everyone drunk, government leaders just gave time off for this long period.

It was during these somewhat slow times that NGO aid leaders in Malawi were invited to attend a gala evening at the home of the United States Ambassador to Malawi. The ADRA Director and I were pleased to accept this invitation and drove the 200 miles to arrive there, thinking we would be among complete strangers. With beautiful American music filling the air; and food and drink delicacies in abundance, we found we were in crowded rooms with many of the Malawi Ministry of Health leaders with whom we had been meeting on behalf of our Child Survival Project in the south. Dr. Louis Sullivan, the U.S. Secretary for Health and Human Services was the guest of honor who spoke to everyone in support of various nations' development services for Malawi. Then I felt a gentle tap on my shoulder! It was a great surprise to be greeted by one of my dear old friends from my days in public health service for Idaho. Dr. James Mason, formerly the Director of Utah's public health services, and at that time the Director for the U.S. Centers for Disease Control in Atlanta, Georgia, wrapped me up in a big hug and said, "What's a nice lady like you doing in a place like this?" Of course, I gave him a delighted, brief answer and he seemed amazed that anyone would spend their 65th year away from home to attempt the awesome challenge of changing lives under Malawi's conditions. That exciting evening and the encouragement I received from my old friend, James, gave me a renewed sense of energy and purpose.

Housing for Two Izungus

Then we sought housing for our two years ahead. Americans already in Malawi assured us that we would not want to live in the lower Shire River Valley, due to the extreme heat and humidity. After all, missionaries, refugee relief workers, European and American NGO aid agencies all headquartered in either the capitol city, Lilongwe, or the commercial capitol, Blantyre. After visiting the Shire Valley, and driving the dusty and rocky trails of the East Bank of the River; then traversing the Mavdbe Game Preserve to find the most remote villages of the West Bank. We were convinced that the only way the Child Survival Project could teach the people and influence positive change in their behaviors, would be for us to live among them. We felt that we must recruit the trainees from within the very villages we would serve. Especially the most neglected villages of Nsanje District.

How often during my years of nursing service, I have read and considered a certain passage in a wonderful book entitled, <u>The Ministry of Healing</u>, by Ellen G. White:

> "Christ's method alone will give true success in reaching the people. The Savior mingled with men as one who desired their good. He showed His sympathy for them, ministered to their needs, and won their confidence. Then he bade them, "Follow me."

There is no question that we would miss the cool climate of Blantyre's highlands, the modern and efficient little upstairs flat with the crows on the roof deck in tuxedos, the two super-markets in walking distance, daily fellowship with other Americans and Europeans, as well as fellowship with the best and brightest of Malawians. Nevertheless, to change a community, an entire valley of hundreds of villages, we needed to follow the Master's model.

About two miles away from the Leprosy Clinic in "beautiful downtown Ngabu" was the squalid, run-down, government hospital There seemed to be very little medical know-how there, although native nurses did the best they could until a visit from a traveling doctor or medical assistant happened. Certainly, there were no physicians based at the hospital or at the Leprosy Clinic. Malamulo Hospital (about 70 kilometers distant) had recently begun to send a team of physicians and nurses to Ngabu once a month to provide continuing education to the Medical Assistants, examine difficult and high-risk patients, perform tubal legations and/or vasectomies, and to expand the teaching of family planning and AIDS prevention.

Beautiful downtown Ngabu was always an exclamation point in our day's adventures, no matter what our business there. Typical, flat roofed, four-post fronts on cement block buildings with corrugated iron roofs, faced the wide black dirt roads that over the many years were navigable by only foot traffic, bicycles, motorcycles and trucks with 4-wheel drive because of huge holes and ruts everywhere. There was no "lay-out" to the town. It had emerged to meet needs of people who beat the barefoot paths from where they settled nearby to the government agency regional headquarters there and the great farming land in that part of the Shire valley. Businesses included the Malawi Post Office, a government hospital, a general store for groceries, household items, a fabric shop, and a few tailors. Their treadle sewing machines on raised porches were often on the porches of other businesses. In addition other businesses included a building supply house, a blacksmith shop, a carpenter shop, a service station, an open-air butcher shop, a police station, schools, four bars, and the Miriwa restaurant.

This restaurant was on the corner where three other roads/trails intersected and right beside what Ken and I decided was the world's largest muddy pothole. Mr. Miriwa and one of his wives opened the restaurant early every morning serving hot rice porridge, eggs and meat with or without the white maize staple, *nsima*, and plenty of strong Malawi tea or coffee. The menus for the day did not vary much from the above, except to occasionally offer a couple of kinds of sandwiches. When we met with village leaders and even with our Advisory Committee (once each month), Mr. Miriwa was happy to serve us. Except for the perpetual Malawi flies, an occasional mosquito and a wandering African brown dog, the premises were kept clean and the food sanitary enough for us *izungus*. The restaurant was shaded parts of the day by a huge tree and one day we saw something strange about that tree from a distance. There were enormous, hulking birds on several branches high in the tree. Some had their long necks tucked under wings as we came closer, then with the sound of the Toyota, they shook themselves awake, and one or two took off in a circling flight. These turned out to be migrating storks that rest awhile in beautiful downtown Ngabu after their long flight from the North. We enjoyed watching them for a few days and again the next year when they returned.

Of course, it was a bit messy under that tree for those few days, but nobody seemed to mind

Behind Miriwa's restaurant and rest house/brothel, the village public market sprawled on the rises of ground under more trees. Individual vendors purveyed their wares that included home-baked "grease balls" – sort of like American doughnut-holes. Considered a delicacy, they fry them in oil, and then put sugar on top. Handmade baskets and children's clothing, along with vegetables, fruits, pineapples, mangos; providing they be in season. Wood carvers showed their primitive art – often done well with a broken Coke bottle. Steel carving tools were beyond their budget! Farmers with a few chickens to sell from their cages made a river of reeds. Sometimes a goat or a pig would be for sale, and the local "medicine man" with various roots and herbs, would create his prescriptions without the FDA interference! Shade-tree markets began at dawn and many stayed until that evening with their oil lamps or wood fires burning to light the villagers to their materials for sale. This was the best place for us to obtain fresh fruits that we always enjoy when we take the trip to the Ngabu market.

Under another tree on another trail, sat the Tinsmith who created many useful tools from sheets of tin and even from the corrugated iron roofing sheets. He used a steel mallet against a heavy piece of iron to create everything from cooking pots to water buckets and lanterns. Adjacent to the Tinsmith was the butcher shop where cattle, goats, pigs, and chickens were slaughtered and hung on the tree to "age." These delicacies could be purchased for the Malawi meal of nsima and relish (stew) when the family could afford it. We were glad to be near-vegetarians who did not need to have meat in our diet. Sometimes in Malawi, we enjoyed the frozen Chambo, a bass-like fish from the lake that we purchased from a Greek man who processed these fish in sanitary ways.

Near one of the entrances to the town, the building

supply house was located. Trucks arrived several times a week from Blantyre loaded with iron sheets, timbers, windows, and very often bags of cement. It was interesting to see how these materials were handled. Although the truck could have backed up to a loading dock, it usually stopped at the roadside and *bambos* would appear from seemingly nowhere to grab the 94-pound bags of cement one by one, place the bag, which they called a "pocket", on their heads and carry it up several steps to the loading dock and into the warehouse. This custom was the protocol that provided work to some young men and they earned a few *tambalas* for their efforts.

Mr. Miriwa insisted that he was a Seventh-day Adventist Christian, yet he and his wife operated another thriving business as a rest-house brothel that mainly served truckers and offered clean showers. Smiling, Mr. Miriwa told us that one of his several wives stayed on their "very good farm" at Makwasa near Malamulo Hospital. The hospital purchased beans and maize meal from his wife there, as well as eggs from her chickens. We never did learn just how many wives Mr. Miriwa had, and he never did show up at the Ngabu S.D.A. church where we attended regularly!

As we made known our need for housing for ourselves, just about everybody we talked to had ideas. The Director of the Leprosy Clinic, Mr. Percival Katumbi (he, himself, a cured leper) suggested that ADRA negotiate with the government to obtain property next door to the clinic and build a quality brick home. This part of the Ngabu community was very high density housing made up of closely spaced, two-room brick houses with tin roofs, sanitary latrines, and small gardens with pigs, chickens, and goats roaming free. The proximity to our office and the visibility we would have to the people were good reasons to consider this possibility.

Other people took us to see vacant African houses:

some with the roofs blown away; some with the cement floors eroded away and chickens dusting themselves in the deep pits in the floors.

At one point we and ADRA-Malawi considered purchasing a lot in the up-scale, low density subdivision that a development group from Germany had begun as a demonstration of "planned community" for the local government. We were pleased with the idea to clear the jungle away from two or three hectares of virgin land, lay out and design a neat little two-bedroom house for us and future ADRA workers to use. We had heard many stories of Malawi's snake infested jungles and had even seen a large green mamba snake in the yard of the Blantyre Adventist Hospital Administrator's home in uptown Blantyre! Therefore, I asked Mr. Phiri as I cautiously pressed my way through the tangle of vines and thorn trees, "Do you ever see any snakes here?" He grinned and said, "Yes, this is their home. We occasionally see the spitting cobra and occasionally a puff adder. Frequently, we see a black or green mamba. They really don't like people very much, and our chickens and pigs help keep them away." I felt my sweaty hair stand up a bit as he so casually informed me about managing snakes, to say nothing of my increased caution as we made our way through that plot of ground with its ancient, virgin jungle intact, serving as home to all kinds of creeping, crawling things. However, I reminded myself that our home, far away in Idaho, is built where there are great dens of timber rattlesnakes, and our presence and the large dog seem to have moved most of them away. The Lord had brought us this far. Surely, He would keep us from these deadly enemies so we could be His feet, His hands, and His great Heart of love reaching out to these precious people. He affirmed me as I considered some of the dangers, recalling to my mind that these people are "the least of these" who lived in such murky ignorance, and yet they longed for something better for themselves and their children.

With the aid of young designers and engineers at the Regional Ministry of Agriculture, we selected the piece of jungle land site and a set of plans already on file with the Director for Agricultural Development (ADD). Just before the contract was signed, we received word that we could not have the lot we had chosen. The ADD was not sure that he wanted to sell any hectares in the subdivision, and that if ADRA were to purchase and build, the government of Malawi could assume ownership and occupancy at any time it chose, canceling any contract. That door to a place for us was slammed shut, but oh, so gently and with the "kindest of intentions" by the current ADD. He went so far as to say that probably the government would never cancel the sale of land, but we needed to be aware that it could!

One house that we considered quite seriously was built for the principal of the Ngabu Training Center, a government hostel where large groups could be trained. There was just one reason why the principal did not live there. Every rainy season (December through February), the river overflowed its banks and sent a flood right through the entire house! We thought it might be possible to build a three-foot high earth and rock barrier to hold back the flood, and one of the government engineers thought so too. Since the house was available rent-free, with Jessie and other local churchwomen's help, we began a clean-up campaign on the house and yard.

As is the African custom, there was no kitchen in the house, but a separate small house in back sheltered space for an electric stove right beside stones on the cement floor to contain an open fire. This fire was for cooking nsima, the thick white maize meal that is the staple of the people, eaten twice a day with some sort of sauce or stew substance that they call "relish". The interior of this brick kitchen-house was well blackened with soot from the fires and there was no evidence that an electric stove had ever been in place. The large entry was not made for a door to be hung, but stood open to the elements and the chickens, pigs and goats! This open kitchen provided enough shelter and air for the fire on the floor to cook well in any weather!

The flush toilet was housed in a separate cubicle adjoining the kitchen, but was cracked and filthy. Adjoining this was the shower room with water piped in but no showerhead or handles. Both of these rooms were complete with doors!

The house, itself, had about two inches of dried mud on all of the floors, with the high water mark about one foot up the walls. Most of the windows were broken and there were no screens. Up until this time, mosquitoes had not been much of a problem. Nevertheless, here, no matter what time of day or night we visited the premises, we were slapping and swatting mosquitoes as they homed in on their warm blood feast from the swampy river area a few hundred feet away. No amount of repellent seemed to deter these determined and vicious droning monsters. We noticed that the nearby mud, brick, and thatch homes often had burning cow dung in their doorways to decrease mosquito interest.

Just when doubt was trying to invade my mind about the possibilities of this house ever becoming habitable for us two “izungus”, our international medical advisor, Dr. Willie, arrived to critique our early planning and guide as he could from his vast experience in several developing countries. He examined our potential house even as the crew was cleaning it, and felt that with just a few kwachas for electrical and plumbing supplies, window screens, cleaning, some furniture, and appliances, and a flood control ditch and dam, we could live quite well. Just as he gave us this positive assessment of possibilities, the mosquitoes stormed him! So I sprayed him and Ken and myself with the last of our American-made DEET formula, picked up my courage from the bottom of the swamp, and told the Lord in my prayers that night that if He wanted us to live there, He'd have to put a plague on the mosquitoes. I thought I could handle everything else.

The next day, we received a message at the Ngabu Tourism Resthouse that had become our home. We were to contact the local Member of Parliament, Mr. Thomas Phinda, who had a modern house under construction that we might lease. The gracious Mr. Phinda seemed very happy to see us, showed us the fine African-style, three-bedroom house with indoor kitchen and two bathrooms indoors! Construction was still just brick walls on cement floors. It needed everything done to finish it, including tin roof, drywalls, and paint, windows, plumbing, electrical, and fencing. Mr. Phinda was frankly out of money with which to finish his "dream home." Would we take it on, complete the construction with the guidance of his construction engineer, Mr. Phiri? He told us that whatever the cost, it could be pro-rated ahead to cover reasonable monthly lease payments, and that ADRA could use the house as long as the agency needed it after we fulfilled our commitment. His traditional home was only a stone's throw from the Principal's house on the edge of the swamp and he was quite sure that we could not be healthy there. He told us that we must not continue to renew that old house, for it is so moist there that everything soon mildews, and that the mosquito scourge cannot be controlled because of the vastness of the Shire River swamps. Not all of the mosquitoes are Anopheles-types that carry the malaria parasite, but many of them are, and we began to see first-hand why the leading cause of death in children, age zero to five, in that country is still Malaria. Mr. Phinda had lost babies to Malaria, and everywhere we went, every day, someone was ill from Malaria.

Children who do survive Malaria may eventually have a decreased sensitivity to the parasites' life cycle in their bodies, and may have what we Americans call only mild "flu-like symptoms" throughout their lives as the recurring bouts of Malaria strike them. That is sometimes true until old age when Malaria again tortures and kills the infected elderly. At that time, the average life span of a Malawian male was only 47 years due to the high death rates for young children and the elderly.

When the ADRA Malawi Director met with the ADRA-Malawi Board of Directors and heard Mr. Phinda's proposal for current and future housing for ADRA Program Managers in Ngabu, versus the only other alternative we could see, they voted to contract with Mr. Phinda. The contracting was left to us, and with wise guidance and materials and costs outlined by Mr. Ndalama Phiri, construction began. Mr. and Mrs. Phinda chose the color scheme and we chuckled at the exterior cobalt blue walls with burnt brick, orange trim! Another African phenomenon even in these new, modern homes is the size of the kitchen versus the size of the separate (from the toilet area) showering room. Our kitchen was ten feet square and had no cupboard space and no window. All supplies must be kept in the pantry adjacent, which had a high window! The showering room was twelve feet wide and sixteen feet long -- big enough for the whole neighborhood to shower together!

It was seven months later when we finally moved from the upstairs flat in Blantyre into this lovely new home that adjoined a thatched-roof, mud hut village, on dry dusty Saopa Road several miles from the swamp. Saopa Road was highly traveled by lorries and heavy truck traffic, delivering people, and supplies to the Mozambiquean refugee camp about eight kilometers beyond us. Dust hung heavy on a breezeless, humid evening, but the mosquitoes were few.

We had been in Malawi for almost one year already, before we could take up residence close to the people we were serving! Most weeks, we simply lived at the Resthouse from our suitcases, traveling almost a hundred miles home to the flat to do laundry and shop for essentials. What a joyous relief it was to find simple furnishings, set up our own washer and dryer, and hook up the air conditioner in the window of our bedroom. Roger had wisely encouraged us to ship these items with us, as well as our computer. Little did we realize what a pleasure it was to have these conveniences while we invested ourselves so heavily in twelve-to-sixteen hour days to put this wonderful project in place and begin to make a difference.

The Office and The Angel

There was no problem in locating modern office space in a part of the Leprosy Clinic in Ngabu. Ngabu is a regional government headquarters especially for the Ministries of Agriculture and Social Services. It was also the last outpost nearest to Nsanje District that has dependable electrical power and, most of the time, potable-piped water.

Our office was one room approximately thirty feet by sixteen feet. Plenty of louvered and screened windows gave a cheery and open feeling to the room, and a ceiling fan was a lifesaver on some of those hot, breathless days. Just outside was a pleasant breezeway with numerous trees of various kinds. Next door were flush toilets and a standpipe with faucet for drinking water. The property owner was actually the Administrator at Malamulo Hospital, located about fifty miles away. The Leprosy Clinic was a branch of that hospital. Our lease payments for the initial three years of the project seemed to be the property owner's answer to prayer. These unanticipated funds would allow a health-care dream of his to come true. This Leprosy Clinic had largely done its work in stamping out leprosy as a public health threat in southern Malawi. The clinic and its well-qualified Medical Assistants needed to expand their sights to provide full primary care services, including a birthing center for high-risk mothers.

We contracted with a fine wood craftsman who was the son of the Leprosy Clinic Director to construct office furniture to meet our requirements: an executive desk, bookshelves, and a conference table with eight chairs. The only problem was that we paid him the money for the cost of the raw materials in advance - up front - and the furniture maker turned out to be a very sick alcoholic. He stayed sober long enough to build a beautiful desk to our specifications, he delivered it and we never saw him again. He was living at home with his parents when we contracted with him, but he completely disappeared, never to be heard from again. We learned more about the Malawi social support system. The adult Malawian will never tell you the "bad truth" about another person. He or she will tell you what he knows you want to hear, always giving his friend, or his son in this case, the benefit of the doubt. This father knew what a beautiful craftsman his son was; he also knew that he was a drunkard. He knew our need and willingness to help local business people by trading with them, and he wanted to believe that this time his son could stay sober and perhaps still find himself by doing good work for us. When we finally realized that this beautiful young man would not deliver, we purchased the rest of the items from a cabinetmaker in Bangula who owned his shop and showed evidence that he could deliver!

I shall never forget the most poignant experience I had my very first day in the Child Survival Office at the Talres Leprosy Clinic. Late in the afternoon, when all the clinic staff had already gone home, I was setting up my personal computer I had brought from home. Using temporary space on a table and a straight chair until appropriate furniture would be delivered, I suddenly heard high pitched wailing outside. I left the office, and there in a crumpled heap on the brick patio was a human figure, shaking all over and wailing in pain. I stooped down to discover a woman who I believed to be about 30 years old, barely covered in rags, her hair disheveled and dirty, and bleeding sores on both her feet. She made motions with her hands to indicate that she was very hungry, so I rushed to my tiny refrigerator to obtain a cup of cold water and a few biscuits for her to eat. She gulped the water alternately with the sweet biscuits while I considered what to do. I decided to run to Rhoda's home only about 200 feet distant and ask her to come and interpret for both of us.

We learned that she was a Mozambiquean refugee from the civil war going on just over the border about 12 miles away. She had known for years that she had leprosy but during the war there was very little medical care available. She told us that her husband and two sons were both killed by the "Renamo" bandits as they plundered her village, but she had hidden and escaped the massacre. She had heard about Talres Lepresy Clinic in Ngabu, so determined that she would walk and walk until she found the clinic. She had been walking and running through the jungle from 'way beyond the border and when she had come upon villages where she thought she might find food, water and rest, she was usually chased away. Rhoda and I washed her face, hands and feet and wrapped the oozing sores on her feet with clean cloth bandages from Rhoda's home. Then we helped the very grateful woman into the project vehicle and took her to the government hospital about 2 miles away in Ngabu *boma*. We knew that she could at least have a cot, water and some food there and transport to the clinic the next day. We learned that she indeed showed up at the clinic, was started on appropriate medicines and taken to live temporarily with an elderly widow woman nearby, who had been healed of leprosy. The women of the local church would see that there was enough food and water for both of the women. For me, this was a most touching experience that reminded me that God had brought me here to minister to "the least of these".

We discovered that the office, while partially

unfurnished, could serve well as a classroom also. Unused benches were available from the clinic next door and we used these benches for seating to train our HSAs. This classroom continued to be an important gathering place after the HSAs were certified and deployed into full service, whenever we brought them together for continuing education and conferencing.

We needed to post a sign about the ADRA Child Survival Project so we could be found in Ngabu. The Leprosy Clinic gave permission for our sign to be made the same size as the Clinic sign and hung on the existing post near the tarmac highway junction with Saopa Road at Ngabu. We had a beautiful enameled metal sign made in Blantyre. It was getting dark one evening when Ken (with his left wrist in a plaster cast after wrist surgery on Christmas Day) finally got to that corner, driving the rented Toyota Hilux pickup, with his power drill, screw driver, nuts, bolts and the sign. As he set about, somewhat clumsily, to attach the sign to the metal post, a voice from the darkness said, "Can I help?" By that time, Ken needed his "torch" (what Malawians call a flashlight) and as he shone it, there was this smiling black face, he said, "Sure." Without many words, this stranger deftly assisted in hanging the sign, utterly fascinated with the power drill that made the holes and drove in the heavy screws. With appreciation, Ken said goodnight to this good stranger and went on his way home to Blantyre (about a three-hour drive in the darkness on pot-holed tarmac, with people walking everywhere).

Three days later, Ken needed to go to a distant village where he had never been. He had received word that we could help with construction of a shallow well there, where the people were walking ten kilometers to obtain river water. He was not even sure how to find this village, but he was on his way when he was flagged by a waving arm and a smiling face at the roadside. It was the same smiling stranger who had helped with the sign. Ken stopped, the man got in the cab and asked where Ken might be going. Ken told him he was on his way to a certain village but he did not know how to find it, nor did he know anyone there. It was so remote that he wondered if there would be anyone who could speak and understand English. The stranger (now a friend) introduced himself as Akim, and said that he had needed a ride to that very village. He said he knew everyone in that village and they do not know much English, but that if he could go with Ken he would be happy to interpret! Then he said, "You know, I speak five languages: Chichewa, Sena, Portuguese, English and the Word of God! I am the pastor of the Ngabu Church of God." Ken began to wonder if Akim was really an angel of the Lord in disguise, because he was right there when he needed him two times. At least he had to have been sent by the Lord, and Ken told Akim so. They had a great day together, meeting with the village chief with Akim interpreting. This was the beginning of a fine friendship. It was quite a touching experience for Ken and he could hardly wait to tell me about it that night.

A few days later, I was driving the Toyota Hilux, just about to leave the grounds of the Ngabu headquarters of the Director for Agricultural Development when a smiling man rode up on his bicycle to my open window and said, "Madam, you don't know me, but we are friends! Muli bwanji? (How are you?)" I knew that this must be Akim and said so, along with "Indili bwino, zikomo" (I'm fine, thank you) offering my hand in a polite handshake out the window, acknowledging that if he was Akim, then surely we are friends! He asked where I was going, and as it happened, I was going to find my way to a possible residence that might be for rent. He said, "Let me go with you because I know the road there!" I quickly agreed and he put his bike in the back of the pickup and joined me in the cab. He knew exactly where to go driving down a dusty foot trail to a bamboo and mud hut that we surely could rent. When I had said "Yes" to the call to Malawi, I had envisioned just such a hut for me, the widow lady missionary. However, we learned that it was already rented. Whew!

Akim told me more about himself. He said that he and his wife, Farmessa, had two children. They lived in Chideu Village where the people were building a mud-brick and bamboo church. He showed me the little mud-brick church with its thatch roof on the edge of Ngabu. It was only about twenty feet square, with a little low, narrow opening for a door that could keep the roving cows out. He asked me about my religion, for he knew that the A in ADRA means Adventist and that means that "You pray on the 7th day."

Time and time again, when Ken or I needed help, or directions, or an introduction somewhere, Akim showed up. We still wonder if that man of God might be an angel!

Recruiting the Project Staff

We encountered the "good truth – bad truth" dynamic again when we were seeking our lead workers for the project. The project territory was to be divided into segments: all the underserved and high-risk villages on each bank of the Shire River would about equally divide the HSAs into two teams, each to be led by a University-prepared Health Inspector. Health Inspectors (HI) are educated much the same as Medical Assistants, but their focus is not on clinical medicine. Theirs is the public health approach to prevention and treatment. They are adept at assessing an entire village or the entire district full of villages as to health risks and the appropriate interventions and/or health education. They understand aseptic technique and can give immunization injections just as well as they can put in a shallow well or other protected water supply. They understand the disease process, nutrition and health, and lifestyle health-illness connections. By design, they are the usual supervisors of the midlevel village health worker, the Health Surveillance Assistant (HSA).

To accomplish the goals of the Child Survival Project, we needed to employ two Health Inspectors (HIs) and one University prepared Horticulturist to carry out the "kitchen gardening" project. We received over forty applications for the HIs and over two hundred applications for Horticulturist! With some help of the ADRA Director, I did a paper screen of the applicants, preparing the short list of candidates. Every application was accompanied by several glowing letters of recommendation, along with a list of several other references to contact. Using carefully worded questions, I contacted the references and to a person, they all gave superlative recommendations for the candidates. We devised both written and oral board examinations that were intended to separate the superb candidates (those who "walked on water") from the good candidates (those who only "drank the water" or maybe could only "pass some water")!

The review board people considered each candidate very carefully for signs and symptoms of Malawi's greatest social disease, alcoholism and its concurrent relational problems. When we finally selected two stellar personalities, both men (nobody in Malawi had heard of a woman Health Inspector yet!) we felt quite sure that we had the very best in committed, energetic, happy, outgoing, teacher-leader-supervisors for the HSAs who were still to be recruited. Rex Mauluka and James Lusuntha, Health Inspectors (HIs) were eager and ready to meet the challenge of this new kind of public health program that could change their nation if just one generation of young families could participate. In this same process, we recruited a fully qualified Horticulturist, Mr. Davis Mchawa, who had just entered "mandatory retirement" after 20 years of service with the Malawi Agricultural Development Agency, Still in his thirties, he had several children who would need excellent education. His family's needs kept him highly motivated as he energetically pursued developing demonstration "kitchen gardens" in the villages we would serve. He would actually be changing the diet so deficient in vegetables to one rich in Vitamins A and C for which most children were sorely lacking. It was not long before Davis became known throughout the Nsanje District as the "Can-Do-Man" for his contagious enthusiasm.

At the same time we recruited the three professional leaders, we advertised in the national press for HSA candidates, and word was spread by the jungle drums throughout the villages in the district. For these 24 paid, student positions, we received over 400 letters of application. The letters that were barely readable were screened out immediately. Individuals who were personally nominated by their pastors of any church denomination were screened into the first short list of approximately forty people. We were amazed when most of our potential candidates turned out to be men! We thought we were recruiting for mostly women who would serve as "village mother-visitors." Our criteria for entry into the program included having completed Standard Eight (US 8th grade) and the ability to read, write and speak both English and their native language of Chichewa. What we had forgotten, is that most little girls who lived in the Nsanje bush, were not sent to school at all. Just a few years ago, there were just a few adult women who could read and write in their own language, Chichewa. Although the schools are required to teach English, it is considered a second language in every grade for over twenty years. The Chichewa language literacy test became our most important screening tool, for many Standard Eight graduates had lived in their own educationally challenged villages where thirty or forty words got them through the day, and what skills they had upon completion of that last year in school had long been forgotten. We were amazed!

We used a different review board for the final short-listed candidates that spread the responsibility outside of

ADRA to include a Masters prepared woman Horticulturist, a government Training Specialist, the local government Health Inspector, the Medical Assistant Director of the Leprosy Clinic and myself. Abiding by the strict employment rules of the Malawi government along with similar rules of the US, we used great care in avoiding invasion of privacy and/or discrimination against race, religion, age, or sex. When the process was finished, we were well pleased with the eleven women and thirteen men, whom became our HSA trainees, and ultimately were deployed to serve in some of the poorest villages. Many of these people came from the poorest of the poor villages; others were from rather well to do homes, but were committed to a life of service for their own people.

Early upon our arrival, we reserved the Ngabu Government Training Center with its dormitories, modern toilet and bathing facilities, food service equipment and teaching halls. This center would serve our purposes for training very well. Except for their testing and interviewing, many of the trainees had never been away from their own village overnight in all of their lifetimes. The Ngabu Training Center was to become their home for nine weeks. They seemed excited to consider themselves pioneers in bettering their villages.

Each of the supervisors were provided with a place to live in their work area, a new yellow Suzuki Agriculture model motorcycle and helmet, all their office supplies, and the government scale monthly salary. Each HSA was provided with a new Raja bicycle, a place to live, working supplies, and their government scale salary. At least half of the HSAs had never held a paying job before, so this employer-employee relationship idea was entirely new to them.

Before our volunteer time was finished, as we were preparing to return home to Idaho, we were greatly saddened to have proof that both of these wonderful college-prepared Health Inspectors were closet alcoholics even at the time we hired them. In addition, one was already infected with AIDS and has since wasted away and died. Fortunately, their diseases were not far enough advanced to prevent their assistance in the training and ultimate deployment of the HSAs.

An Advisory Committee and the "DIP"

In between expeditions to explore African style housing, we conducted staff and trainee recruitment. Somehow, we held to the time frames we had set for planning and beginning the Child Survival Project. With the necessary research done on the population we would serve, I could write the USAID-required "Detailed Implementation Plan" (DIP) and send it to Washington, DC, for approval by both ADRA International and USAID. In addition, I had begun to get acquainted with national, regional, and local district public health officials. We were impressed with the physicians in lead roles who were nearly all from The Netherlands. It seems that for young people to study medicine in The Netherlands, they must first commit to serve at least two years in a third world developing country upon graduation. To a person, these were delightful people, hard working, bright clinicians who also were intensely committed to making a difference in the health circumstances of this nation, as they served "their time" in Malawi. Most of the rest of the staff in the bureaucracy, and certainly those out in the local hospitals, clinics, and health posts were national Malawians. Their schooling was at the University of Malawi, or at one of the small private hospitals, such as at the Catholic Trinity Hospital in Muona on the East Bank of the Lower Shire River, or at the one-hundred years old, Seventh-day Adventist, Malamulo Hospital, in Thyolo District, about 70 kilometers southeast of Blantyre in a very rural, bush environment..

As I met with public health leaders in the Ministry of Health, they were always gracious in giving me their time and attention. They described to me the system in place to render public health services, but the extreme shortage of funds had rendered the system impotent to deal with anything beyond central community needs. I learned from them that vast areas of Malawi had no health teacher or health outpost. These same areas had low literacy rates and very high death rates due to rampant preventable diseases such as malaria, AIDS, cholera, diarrhea, measles, tuberculosis, and pneumonia. I listened intently, making many notes. I asked questions about our target area: the hot, fertile, steaming Nsanje District. Moreover, I listened intently as they told me their concerns and interests. When I made known to them the project objectives and asked for their support, they offered the resources they had. These included colorful posters and pamphlets with simple but important health messages addressing the rampant problems. I learned that we could purchase medicines and supplies at government rates when the project would be approved by the District Health Officer. There would be no charge for certain audio-visual equipment and materials they would loan to us, as we needed them. Most of the goods and equipment available to us had been provided to the Malawi Ministry of Health by donor organizations such as UNICEF, Save The Children, World Vision, and The World Health Organization. Malawi had neither the personnel nor the funds at that time to use these excellent supplies. These early visits generated formal and informal partnerships that became the strength of the program, for early suspicions were laid aside and trust grew as we opened and shared ideas with these wonderful, knowledgeable people.

As the DIP was nearing completion, I shared draft copies of it with some of these health professionals, asking for their feedback. They helped me to set realistic objectives and to plan strategies to bring new health knowledge to thousands of people in neglected ignorance. When I asked some of these new friends to serve on our Child Survival Advisory

Committee (CSAC), they were eager to do so. The membership of the CSAC included twelve officials, representing their areas of authority and expertise. including Regional Health Officer, his Maternal/Child Health Nurse, the Nsanje District Health Officer, local pastors, and representatives from the local Catholic hospitals and clinics in Nsanje District where over 750,000 people live. I held a high degree of respect for each member's vast experience, cultural knowledge, and medical/social wisdom. The advisory committee met once a month in various venues somewhere in the bush in our target areas. CSAC helped to finalize the DIPand set the standards for the village door-to-door survey of current village health knowledge, attitudes and practices. Hearing the reports and motivating us with their coaching encouraged us. Members of this committee helped us to open the right doors to the social, religious, and political leaders of Nsanje District villages. They introduced me to similar project leaders in Child Survival located in other Districts across the nation. These leaders were sponsored by other NGOs, including World Vision, Save The Children, ADRA, and of course the International Eye Foundation. As we came together as a group of NGO leaders, we developed into a vital network of energetic project managers. We supported one another, shared methods and unique approaches to the common problems we faced every day and sometimes were able to influence public health policy in the nation.

The rapport and synergism within this committee was unique in that problem solving and decision-making was by consensus. At the close of each meeting, there was much satisfaction as we evaluated the month's challenges and opportunities and laid plans for months ahead. As is the Malawi national custom, we opened each meeting with prayer, traveled to various sites in the bush, ate together, and looked forward to future working sessions.

CHAPTER 4

The Process For Positive Change

One Life at a Time

OUr CSAC recommended that the Knowledge, Attitudes, and Practices (KAP) study be contracted out to the Social Sciences Department of Chancellor College at Zomba. Chancellor is a part of the University of Malawi system, but is the oldest campus in the country and located in the beautiful, former colonial capitol city of Zomba about fifty kilometers north of Blantyre. When I contacted him, the department director was most cordial and eager to participate. Any reasonable way to generate additional funds for his department appealed to him. He showed us similar successful studies his research assistants and graduate students had performed. Then we went over the basic design, the elements, and standards for the study, and met the student who would be assigned to our work, and we signed the contract.

The plan was for us to find one hundred volunteers from the project area, bring them to the Ngabu Training Center in two groups of fifty where they would be trained by our graduate college student for one week. They would learn and practice the methods and skills of door-to-door interviews, using the fifteen-questions in simplest Chichewa terms, and recording the answers on a separate sheet for each household. The actual survey was expected to take about four weeks, with volunteers, supervised by the student researcher, working in their territories four or five days each week.

The project was responsible for transporting the surveyors to and from their daily locales, while the researcher, Mr. Nkoma, was responsible for quality control and supervision of the volunteer team leaders. We had two college students for drivers of rented transport vehicles that would carry the women surveyors to their assigned villages, day by day. One driver was from Capetown, South Africa, and the other was from the United States. They were happy to get involved in this activity. Everything seemed to be falling in place.

To find volunteers to be trained as door-to-door surveyors, I was advised to first contact the Seventh-day Adventist pastors within our project area. There were two of them, each responsible for over twenty separate churches scattered throughout the bush on either side of the river. Pastor Zaccheous and his wife were delighted to participate and assured us that they had at least fifty women who were members of their church women's group, called Dorika, who would be happy to volunteer. We outlined the proposal to them, and later met with representatives of several Dorikas to find their interest. ADRA's gifts to each woman for her participation were to include a waterproof shoulder bag at the beginning of their survey work, and a custom tailored Dorika uniform for each woman at the end of the job well done. The women were excited at the opportunity. The only recruitment criteria were that they would be free to leave their village for one week's training; and be able to work at some distance from their homes for four weeks, returning home for the weekends; and they must be able to read, speak, and write simplest Chichewa.

On the West Bank, we were accompanied by the Adventist Youth Director, Pastor Gabriel Moyo, from church headquarters in Blantyre to help locate the pastor for the area, Jim Nazombe. We had been unable to contact Pastor Nazombe so we just drove toward his home in Phokera. About twenty kilometers before we reached Phokera, on a street typically crowded with lorries, bicycles, people walking, goats, pigs, chickens and cows, Pastor Gabriel spotted Pastor Jim, walking his bicycle! I could never have spotted him, having never seen him before. Nevertheless, even if I had known him, I don't think I would have seen him. Gabriel called to Jim, and delighted to see us, he tossed his bicycle into the pickup, and we completed the drive to his home. Without telephones and with slow, uncertain mail service, it took little miracles like this for us to connect with the right people at the right times.

I was immediately impressed with young pastor Jim's manner and bearing. Bright, articulate and interested, he quickly grasped the goals of our project and wanted very much for his Dorika women to be a part of it. However, his problem was that very few of the Dorika women could read and write their own language. They would be willing, but not capable, to undertake the work of the survey. He said that perhaps he could find two dozen who could. As we had driven the valley roads, we saw at least two Catholic parish headquarters, and several churches that had signs reading, "C.C.A.P.." Therefore, I asked Jim if he knew any of the other pastors. He looked at me, incredulous, answering, "No, you do not understand. I am the only pastor for twenty-seven churches!" I replied, "I mean, do you know the pastors of the other denominations such as the Catholic priest and that C.C.A.P. church?" Again, Jim seemed surprised, but said, "Oh, yes, I know Father Kelly at Kalimba Parish and Pastor Kadzua Banda at the Central Church of Africa, Presbyterian." I asked him if those churches had organized women's groups who do community services as the Dorikas do, and he was quite sure they did, but he was astonished that I would suggest that we might work together with other non-Adventist Christians. Jim agreed to make appointments for him to accompany me to meet with Father Kelly and Pastor Banda one week from that day.

We met Father Kelly puffing on his pipe in his office. He had not yet offered us a chair when he let loose a puff of smoke and asked, "Why, after one hundred years of working side by side here in Malawi, do you Adventists now come to us Catholics and ask for help in health work?" I was taken back with this sudden confrontation, but I remembered my personal commitment to serve as Jesus did, and Jesus gave me the answer: "With all due respect to you and those that have been here before us, I cannot speak to what has happened or not happened in the past. I only know that Jesus is inclusive, not exclusive. If Jesus were here today, He would want all who call themselves by His name to work together on behalf of the poor, the sick, and dying. I think that the women of your church and the women of Adventist churches love and worship the same God and Savior, Jesus Christ. I believe they all would enjoy experiencing the power of the Holy Spirit if they were to come to work together in the name of Jesus Christ, their Savior." The old Irish priest let out another cloud of smoke, and gasped, "Well, I've been right here for over thirty years, and I've never heard anything like this. Raphael, find about twelve women who can read and write to help with this Child Survival thing!" He was red in the face and abruptly excused himself as he left us with Raphael, his Secretary, who gently plied us with questions until he felt he knew us well enough in order to recruit some volunteers. I agreed to meet with whomever he recruited in two weeks from that day to orient them to their venture and learn of any needs or questions they might have.

From that quite exciting experience, we went to meet with Pastor Banda and his wife, Elizabeth,at their humble home. Pastor Banda was most enthusiastic about his members participating in the survey and explained that in his congregation there were also Anglicans and Episcopalians, since there were no churches of those denominations in this part of the lower Shire valley. In a few days, I took my favorite interpreter and guide, Mr. Welton Singano, to meet with Pastor Kadzua Bandas women's group. They sang and danced for joy in the praise of Jesus, their Lord, and Savior, to welcome us and to let us know that they really wanted to serve Him this way.

As a motivational tool, I again shared with both the Catholic and Protestant groups that they would receive the waterproof bags at the beginning of their work, the weeklong training experience in the fairly modern dormitory at Ngabu, and at the end of their work, each one would receive the uniform of their organizations. In both cases, they were quick to respond. "Zikomo, zikomo, for such generosity. The cost of the uniforms is more money than we can earn in one year. As you can see, we cover our bodies with these blouses you Americans send in used clothing bundles, and this square of cloth forms our wrap-around skirt. But we are clean, and happy to be with you, and to help the children in villages where they do not know God or how to stay healthy."

Then the Catholic women's faces clouded over and they said, "Our organization does not use uniforms. What will you give us instead?" We negotiated for beautiful dresses for church wear, so all the nuns and neighbors in church would know that they had done something wonderful for their Lord!

The Presbyterian, Anglican and Episcopal women each needed uniforms. The Presbyterian women wore black and white, the Anglican wore blue and white, and the Episcopal women wore black, blue, and white! The Adventist Dorikas wore maroon and white uniforms. Every group of women began careful measurements of each other and submitted them as guidance for the tailor we would employ to create this beautiful array of uniforms.

In beautiful downtown Ngabu there was one roadside tailor with his treadle sewing machine who was very happy to strike the bargain to create just over 50 uniforms for the groups of church women, , 130 zippered, water-proof bags for the volunteers in the KAP study, the 24 HSAs and a few extra for other helpers. Yes, the men in Malawi are proud to have and use a shoulder bag. Then we contracted with a tailor to set up his sewing machine on our covered office patio, and as the measurements came in, he created the beautiful uniforms. Later the HSAs decided on royal blue for their duty shirts and A-line duty dresses, and our tailor was very happy because he was making more money in six weeks than most tailors earn in five years! In addition, we found a custom sign-maker in Blantyre who created individual identification pins for the "ADRA CHILD SURVIVAL VOLUNTEER" and nametags for the HEALTH SURVEILLANCE ASSISTANTS and the ADRA CHILD SURVIVAL PROGRAM SUPERVISOR. Identity and self-esteem go hand in hand in this culture. Villagers in general, and political and social leaders seem to accept the village worker better with an identity allied to a known service group.

ADRA had become well known in the lower Shire valley when they had provided flood relief to victims of an enormous flood there in 1988. Food, clothing, and blankets had been distributed to hundreds of victims. It was during this relief work that the ADRA Director saw children with "failure-to-thrive" and kwashiorkor disease due to malnutrition. He could see in the eyes of the children and their distraught mothers that many of those children would die in just a few days. ADRA intervention had come too late.

It was then that the Director's aching heart was inspired to appeal to USAID for Child Survival funds.

In order to make them aware of the project and the importance of the survey, we wanted to meet with the village chiefs, and political party coordinators. This would make our door-to-door survey better, by enabling us to target our teaching and interventions to those villages that had the highest risk families. Therefore, we learned from the government Health Inspectors how to get written messages in their languages to hundreds of these village leaders on both sides of the river, setting dates when we would be present under a certain tree, or in a certain school auditorium, to meet with them and invest their interest and approval in what we were about.

For several of these meetings, either Mr. Nkoma or the local manager for an International Eye Foundation project, Mr. Mlozi Banda, served as my travel companion and interpreter. However, for the largest meeting of all, with over 200 village and political leaders present under the giant malumba tree, no interpreter showed up. I had met the Nsanje District Health Inspector (HI) for the East Bank villages, and he was there. I greeted him and asked him to interpret for me. Twelve Muona Dorika women were there in their best chitenjis and a large bamboo mat to sit on. They found a spot right near me, front, and center. In addition, the visiting physician from the USA was with me, Dr. Willie. People seated themselves in a wide semi-circle as they arrived for the meeting, and by that time, I had learned a few words of Chichewa greeting and the little curtsy that Malawians do in greeting. Therefore, while I was waiting for an interpreter, I knew that I could lose nothing by greeting each individual personally with a handshake and a "Muli bwanji" and or a "Mulungu akudalitseni, bambo" which means "God bless you, sir." I could feel the warmth of their acceptance and my anxiety about no interpreter began to fade.

While people continued to arrive from their long walks to get there, I continued the greeting process, showing my joy at seeing the HI arrive. The people clapped when they realized that their HI and I were friends. Therefore, I began my story. I told them that it was the love for God that made me want to come help them to learn better ways so their babies needn't die. I told them that I came not as a "great white bwana" but as their sister who cared for them before I knew them, and that Ken beside me is their brother. Then with wonderful help from the HI interpreting, I described the imminent door-to-door survey with volunteer churchwomen conducting the village visits. I asked for their cooperation. We would provide the volunteers with transportation, but they might need to eat a meal someplace, or have a cup of cold water, or even stay overnight.

Then I described how a village health worker would come to live amid some of them to teach and guide their families into better health. I tried to help them see how precious their children are as the hope of tomorrow when we oldsters would be gone; that good health of the people is good for their beautiful nation and that their President-for-life was happy for this teaching. The political party was more active in the bush villages than in the cities and seemed to be more important than religion or education, so I tried to honor their government whenever I could do so. When I finished my talk, I asked them to talk back to me.

One by one, across the circle, the hospitality talk came back to me, welcoming us and the project, promising that our people would be treated well wherever they went, and hoping that all 3,000 villages on the East Bank could have a health worker living among them! Finally, one very elderly chief haltingly stood to his feet, leaning on his stick, said, "But, sister, tell us when you Americans will bring the magic medicine that will stop 'Edze' (AIDS) from killing our people?" I swallowed hard, hesitated to answer, when a young chief stood up across the circle. Bowing deeply to the elder, he said, "Bambo, there is no magic medicine that will stop *Edze.* We must change our behaviors and how we live in order to stop the killer. No more prostitutes when we are away from our wives. We must teach our children to have only one wife and to have fewer children and to keep the ones we have healthier so we don't need to replace them by weakening our wives through too many birthings." The elder sat down, I bowed deeply in appreciation to both of them and the twelve Dorika women jumped to their feet, saying to me, "Shall we sing our song now?" I nodded assent, and they sang and sang all sixteen verses of the song they had written themselves about how God made one man for one woman and we have ignored His way. One man for one woman is God's way to stop Edze and one man for one woman is what we must begin to do now if we are to save our loved ones. When they finished and sat down, there was a long silence with only the sound of the soft breeze playing in the leaves above. I had no idea that they would sing that song. I had heard it once, but they had come to see and hear what happened that day, and to wait their opportunity to teach in their own way --singing. It was so moving that I had tears in my eyes.

Then I noticed an elderly woman who was beautifully dressed with exotic colors, huge puffed sleeves and a matching turban artfully wrapped on her head. She said that she was the trusted treasurer for the Malawi Congress Party in the District and that she had seen a lot of missionaries come and go but not one like me. "There you are, she said, "with dust on your shoes from walking the trail to the meeting tree, sweat on your face from the afternoon heat and humidity, and tears in your eyes as you were touched by my people's singing." She said, "You say that you come as our sister, and I believe you. I have seen the love in your eyes and in your tears, and in the touch of your hand. Welcome to the rest of your family. We accept you and want to help you in every way to do this good work for our children. Feel free to come and go on our roads, to mingle with us without fear or danger, and whenever we know that you or your Bambo are teaching, we will come. You are most welcome." As she said this to me, she knelt before me, and I could not stand above her, so regardless of their custom of kneeling before their own superiors, I knew I had to kneel to see her face as she spoke. Therefore, I, too, knelt before those hundreds of her kinfolk and wept as she paid me the greatest compliment I have ever received.

Pastor Zaccheus was present, and when I asked him to close this two-hour meeting with a prayer. Only this prayer was without interpretation for me because Zaccheus talked so fast, but many men, and a few women, (Christian, Muslim, and Animist) around that circle were weeping joyfully when he closed in the name of Jesus. In addition, every person there, men and a few women, came and shook my hand as they bowed slightly with hundreds of "Zikomo, Zikomo Kwambiris" – Thank you, thank you so much.

The visiting American physician Dr.Willie and Ken were greatly moved. We were all very tired, sweaty, and dusty and we still must travel another hour facing into the late afternoon's glaring sun to reach our destination for overnight rest. We had made reservations with Raphael, the Catholic priest's secretary, to stay in the hostel at Kalimba Parish. We knew of no other place to stay. As we drove along the pitted tarmac road, darkness had overtaken us and our headlights picked up motion ahead in the road, so Ken slowed to a crawl and we could see partially clothed people scurrying away in the darkness. We had just interrupted the evening bathing time for village women! Even though this stream was not clear and clean, the water was cool and the tarmac was a warm place to dry off and replace the *chitenji* around the body.

When we arrived at the Kalemba Parish gate, Raphael met us to say that a group of nuns had just arrived from out of the bush for a few days' rest and he could not very well allow men into the hostel at the time nuns were sleeping there! What to do? Raphael knew of one small Resthouse that might have a room for us. It was just a few blocks distant in Bangula boma.

The proprietor of the Holiday Resthouse told us that there was just one room left but it had two twin beds. We looked at each other and said, "We'll take it!" There was a shower and flush toilet bathroom attached, but no screens on the windows and mosquitoes were on their way in! While the good doctor took his shower, Ken and I went to find a shop that might be open to purchase the special coils to burn near the windows to keep the mosquitoes out. We found them and returned to find Willie asleep, snoring vigorously while the mosquitoes hummed. Ken chose to shower last, but as he inspected the facilities, he warned me to be careful not to step on the big toad-frog on the floor!

My turn for that delicious shower and guess what? There was no more water. The water tank was just outside this house on a high platform with a ladder. It was filled early every morning by a bucket brigade of young boys who carry the water from the one town well every morning. There was <u>no more running water!</u> Then it struck me -- there must be clean water still in the toilet tank, and yes! -- the tank was full of cool, clean water above the toilet. Therefore, I actually took a bath and enjoyed it, out of the toilet-holding tank! No civilized bath ever felt any better. Yes, the toad stayed out of the way, and I was too weary to let him bother me. As I was drying my weary body, I heard sounds outside and looking out the shower window I could see several boys with water cans, climbing the ladder to the Resthouse water tank! It was dark, but the management had called for more water. And it was delivered promptly, in the light of the moon! And Ken had a wonderful shower!

We collapsed into that narrow, hard, but clean African bed but could not sleep. Truckers were coming back to their rooms from an evening of revelry. Some of them brought girls with them and the shrieks and sounds penetrated to our room. Willie kept right on snoring and slept soundly all night. Every hour Ken got up to light another mosquito coil to keep the ravenous beasts away. Just as we began to doze at about four in the morning, dawn was breaking and the gardener began work -- hoeing weeds in the rocks just outside our open window. Clink, clink, clunk -- there was no more chance for sleep for Ken and me. When the young boys began to whistle and chatter as they climbed up the wooden ladder laden with huge buckets of water to replenish the Resthouse water system, even Willie woke up! So much for sleep, and we laughed as we told him all that had happened while he had snored on. We found a restaurant where we had eaten before and devoured steaming huge bowls of hot rice porridge for breakfast. With a cup of strong Malawian tea to go with our rice, we felt ready to face another day of meetings with other village chiefs.

One of the meetings that next day was with about fifty chiefs, headmen, and MCP officials in a large brick classroom with benches and blackboard. Our interpreter, Mlozi Banda, the local manager for the International Eye Foundation Vitamin A Project, had preceded me with his health instructions relative to Vitamin A and the need to distribute it to all the children in their villages. He gave me a flowery introduction and I followed with my presentation similar to the one the day before. When I asked for their responses, many speeches of appreciation and willingness to cooperate were made. Then the MCP District Counselor stood up -- he was about six feet, six inches, tall (most Malawi men are of moderate height -- very few over five feet, eight inches). With a deep baritone voice he reinforced every positive response before his, and then he said, "If mayi (mother) Jarrell and her bambo can come all the way to us from the United States as volunteers, surely we can not only cooperate with their efforts for our children, we, too, must volunteer to help them and thus to help ourselves." The group gave him resounding applause in affirmation.

At a brief break in the meeting, all the people left the hot brick building for the shade of the trees, the men congregating together and the women sitting together on the other side of the building. Therefore, I followed the women. We smiled at each other, and one of them laid a *chitenji* on the ground for me to sit on, but I could see that none of them spoke or understood English. I knew that they had understood everything I and the visiting American doctor had said because of Mlozi's fine interpretation. I said to them in English with hand motions from my speaking mouth out to the world, "Please tell the other women in your villages what you have heard from me today." They shook their heads. They did not understand. So then, I thought about the "jungle drums" we often jokingly talk about. Ken and I heard them every night and wondered what they were saying across the miles to those who could hear them. Therefore, I placed my hands on the ground as though they were on a drum, beat out a rhythm on the ground, while my voice said, "Bum, butty bum, bum, bum." They laughed and laughed in understanding, as I made hand motions of speaking with my mouth and spreading the word so others could hear. I laughed with them 'till we all had tears in our eyes. I could feel their love and acceptance of me as we stood and they each gave me the typical African woman's handshake (it means the same as a hug!) with palms meeting in an audible "slap" and then a firm squeeze. It was another day where God's love abounded. Moreover, I knew our message about the project would reach many villages. After these two days in the bush with us, Dr. Willie had a pre-evaluation visit that showed him clearly that we were up to the task of teaching and loving these precious primitive people, even as he experienced many of our challenges.

Door-to-Door Dilemmas and Disasters

We chartered busses to go out to the bush byways and pick up fifty women at a time, bring them to Ngabu Training Center for their one week of training by the University researcher and study leader. I could hear them singing gospel songs long before the bus turned into the grounds of the center. They alighted with their small katundu (cloth bundle or basket of their personal goods), and smiles and hugs or warm handshakes for me. They chose their rooms and their roommates. Some with babies brought a ten or twelve-year old girl to serve as nanny during class times. Others set about to find a nanny through the Training Officer at the Center.

Staying a week away from their home villages was a first time experience for most of these women. They had never been out of their villages. They had never seen electric lights, flush toilets, or shower baths. They were ecstatic, and stayed up nearly all night the first few days, just to talk "girl-talk" as they never had before. Rhoda and Jessie from the Ngabu Dorika helped the women organize their own support system considering their potential needs. The women chose one leader who would serve as spiritual leader and problem solver for the week. Each morning at six, Rhoda or Jessie would show up, wishing them "*Chadzuka bwanje*" (Good morning!) and making sure that their questions were answered and basic needs met.

Every evening Rhoda and Jessie came to the Training Center after the evening meal, again to ascertain that all were all right. If any were sick, they were escorted to the government hospital about a block away. Fortunately, nobody became acutely ill during these training times. On Wednesday evenings, the entire membership of Rhoda and Jessie's churchwomen's group, *Dorika*, arrived with their babies on their backs. They came about four o'clock to sing worship songs, pray, read a scripture and praise God for His goodness. Instead of fifty women's voices, there were about seventy-five singing in rich four-part harmony. They were having such a good time that when someone suggested, "Let's take our songs to the market", they formed a curving and weaving line in close formation, singing and chanting praises to *Mulungu* (God).

The evening market is under the trees with vendors sitting on the ground, their wares spread out before them. The women snaked their song-line all through the banana and clothing vendors, over the dry ditch to the bicycle repairman and on, and on, until they had covered the market of "beautiful downtown Ngabu." They were ready to sleep as soon as they said goodnight to the *Dorika* women who must walk the dark, dusty trails to their thatched roof homes as far away as five kilometers.

The next morning, the governmental Director of the local office of the Ministry of Agriculture stopped me on the road to inquire about why our trainees are always singing! I asked him whether he liked the sound or not. He said he had never heard such fine music – there must be some angels singing with them. These beautiful women from Catholic, Presbyterian, Anglican, Lutheran and Adventist backgrounds, found that they were really one, united under the banner of Jesus Christ's love.

Mr. Nkoma showed up and began the training for the survey procedures. He was clearly not a Christian and the songs about Jesus seemed to annoy him. He had little patience with crying babies, or mothers leaving class when the nanny called them. In fact, I felt that he basically did not respect women. Some days he showed up two hours late to start the class. I attended as often as all the other management responsibilities allowed, and I could see that the women, indeed, understood their teacher, learning and practicing the knowledge, skills, and attitudes they must employ to obtain the KAP data. Nevertheless, I knew something was wrong with Mr. Nkoma.

During the teaching of these fifty women, we discovered Mr. Nkoma at our Resthouse, very drunken and with a woman who was not his wife. His wife and children were at home, 150 kilometers distant at Zomba. During this week, Mr. Nkoma was late to the classroom more and more often. When I talked to him about how the class was going, he had all the right answers. As we reviewed the deployment plan and the quality control measures he would take, he seemed to be tracking all right. However, Ken and I both knew that we were dealing with a beautiful young man who was trapped in alcoholism.

At the deployment stage -- the actual beginning of women collecting information from village households – Mr. Nkoma did not follow through to check up on the survey team captains, nor to randomly check the filled-out forms. I did not learn about this important breakdown until the second week, and I promptly found Mr. Nkoma and asked him about it. He said he felt the team leaders were doing a fine job checking at the end of each day and there was no need for his further checking. As he backed off from his quality control responsibilities, the survey women became lax in completing the questionnaires. They found if they asked only a few of the questions they could be finished with each day and their entire territory much sooner. When one of the college student volunteer drivers needed to leave for home in the US, Ken was involved in the transporting of the surveyors. One day he drove the old ADRA ambulance with seats in back over the rocky trails up a steep slope to drop off the surveyors. It took him about two hours to weave his way back down the foot-path trail in the vehicle, and lo and behold!, there were the women he had just dropped off at the top of the mountain that morning. They had beaten the vehicle down the slope and did not realize it, so their embarrassment was acute as Ken discovered them sitting under the trees, filling out forms for imaginary people in the village at the top of the mountain. Ken brought these forms home to me with his hilarious -- but dismaying report. However, it was then and only then that I could believe the worst. The worst was really true. Without supervision and daily checking and feedback from Mr. Nkoma, they had become demoralized and their data was completely useless. A fairy story at best!

Oh, there were the good and faithful volunteers. Nora needed to stay a full week in a remote village, so we sent a few kwachas with her to give to her hosts to cover the nsima and relish she would need for food. She brought her own sleeping mat and an extra chitenji, so she could wash and dry one while wearing the other for a sleeping garment. As she slept in her host's bamboo and mud/thatch hut one night, she was awakened suddenly by a warm body and a nudging against her body. She thought, "What is this?" and in the darkness, she pushed away the family goat that had come in out of the cool night breeze. She laughed and laughed as she told her story of sleeping with a goat!

Lame grandmother Alice Natiya from Bangula trudged many a mile, faithfully gathering her data, turning in her completed forms at the end of a week in the distant bush. She had gone so far away on foot that she discovered a village that was not even shown on the government maps, so she included that one too.

To the women who needed to spend overnight time in distant villages we provided a few kwachas each for their hosts. But, bright and creative, they could see that those kwacha might do more good for everyone if they would take a basket full of sweet potatoes or bananas from their own garden and take that to their hosts while they spent our kwacha on a new chitenji for themselves! We had to overlook some of their child-like games when they stayed true to their ultimate mission.

One day, Ken needed to go to Blantyre and one of the volunteer surveyors asked if she could ride along because her husband worked in Blantyre and she would like to see him. Ken agreed to take her and picked her up in her village. They had not gone far when several people were standing on the roadside waving their hands as if to flag Ken down. Elizabeth shouted, "Stop, Stop, I know those people and we need to give them a ride." Before Ken could reach a full stop, Elizabeth had opened the door. She jumped out of the borrowed Peugeot ambulance, ran around to the rear, and let four people in. In another few miles, this happened again with Ken stopping at her urgent request as she jumped out and ran to the back to let in another four people. This time, Ken could see Elizabeth better in the rear view mirror. She had her hand out and was taking money from each of the new passengers! Then, Ken realized that when a Malawian is waving in that manner they are not only asking for a ride, that hand wave means he or she has kwacha to pay for the ride! Elizabeth said nothing about the money, but she had a pocket-full. She was just making the best of an entrepreneurial opportunity! After all, a girl can't go to the city without

kwacha! Ken enjoyed the joke on him and never brought the subject up, for he would never charge to pick up a friend!

We learned in retrospect that the valid data in the survey should have been entered into the computer on a daily basis by qualified data entry personnel. Those types of services were available, but the ADRA Director felt he could employ some bright junior high school students to enter the data whenever they were free, at less cost. Data entry soon fell apart and ultimately was contracted out to a firm in the capitol city. Because of the poor quality data, the basic KAP study provided very little usable data and the project had to be evaluated in other ways to measure positive changes in knowledge, attitudes, and practices. Therefore, we learned what we should have known even if we had done this same study in the US. The usefulness of survey data is only as good as the level of quality control. The failure of this study was my only disappointment, and that was a big one. And, no, we did not pay Chancellor College for one-third of the agreed upon sum, due to the failure of the quality control obligation by their Mr. Nkoma, whom we eventually learned that at that very time was a very sick alcoholic with AIDS at the age of 24.

Training Trials and Triumphs

Before we completed the process of selecting the 24 trainees for the Health Surveillance Assistant program, we wanted to give every opportunity for likely candidates to emerge from the cadre of volunteers who had served in the Household Survey. We held a "Train the Trainer" workshop at a lovely retreat center near Zomba. Miss Vickie Graham traveled all the way from Washington, DC, to lead in the training, teaching village people to teach other adults in culturally meaningful methods. It was a wonderful week, ending with a kick-off celebration bringing together members of our Advisory Committee and other public health officials to share the Detailed Implementation Plan, to network with leaders in children's services and learn from one another the various supportive roles that neighboring agencies would provide to help the project be a sustainable success.

The highlight of the training of the forty participants (they were the cream of the volunteer surveyors!) was discovering their innate gift for drama. The simple bush person can best learn or teach by action, and with each new health message, these participants could invent a script and act it out dramatically within a half an hour. Next in their natural teaching/learning style came the use of humorous posters that they devised, or that could be obtained from their Ministry of Health.

At the end of the week, the new HI supervisors administered a Chichewa literacy test, both written and oral, and it was heart breaking to see the failures. Only seven of the forty had adequate reading, writing, and speaking skills to participate in the anticipated HSA training. It was my sad task to return the results to each of them privately and to somehow show them that they are loved and needed as role models in their own villages. I encouraged those who had failed, to begin to study their native language as well as English at every opportunity and we gave them books to study from. Their sense of failure was very hard for them and very much so for Miss Vickie and me. It was my privilege, however, to present their uniforms to them and to encourage them to continue to be leaders for good things in their churches and villages. Later, I often saw those who did not enter the HSA training program. They were always happy to see me and tried to tell me how much it meant to them to be involved as far as they had been.

All the participants at the “Train The Trainer” workshop fell in love with fair-haired Miss Vickie. They were not the only ones. Our volunteer driver, Allen, from South Africa, adored her. They were both in late twenties: he, a Christian soldier of fortune; she, an educator par excellence on an adventure in Africa that she had only dreamed of. Therefore, when Miss Vickie expressed her desire to see some of our bush country, Allen was quick to volunteer and they came to Ken and me to see what could be arranged. So far, Miss Vickie had seen only the city of Blantyre and the lovely rural, retreat center. She wanted to see the Lower Shire Valley we had talked about. She wanted to see the all engrossing, shade tree and barroom gambling game of “Bau” (pronounced, “bow”) and learn how to play it; she wanted to sleep under a Baobab Tree under the African stars!

Allen begged to be allowed to take our rented ADRA vehicle to give Miss Vickie her thrill of a lifetime. He promised to be circumspect in every way and to drive safely, taking care of the vehicle and Miss Vickie. In her way,

Vicki's grin and nodding head was begging too! How could we say, "No?" Nevertheless, we made them both promise that this excursion would not be talked about for at least a year, anywhere! We filled the vehicle tank with petrol, Ken checked everything under the hood and placed an extra jerry can of petrol on the bumper. We packed a wonderful lunch for them and a two-gallon jug of water for drinking and sent them down the road, chuckling to ourselves. However, in the back of our minds, if anyone objected to such a use of the project vehicle, or if they should have a wreck, or if someone should think, "Nice young people just don't do that," it would be we who would have to take the consequences. We both knew that we would do the same thing for our own children in a similar circumstance. They were delightful adults.

Being without a vehicle for a week-end gave us a good excuse to just hang out at the government Rest- house in Ngabu, where our basic needs were well met with good meals, a clean and air-conditioned room, pleasant conversation with other guests and the staff, and good walking trails for a bit of exercise. No drive to church, no driving to the office to work away a Sunday as was often my custom, -- just a quiet weekend together.

The two adventurers returned right on schedule, having traveled all the way to the dangerous Mozambique border and back without so much as a flat tire or an argument. Those African stars were in Miss Vicki's eyes and Allen was quietly pleasant. Miss Vickie had just one problem. Allen had tried to ignore the picnic fare in favor of eating at roadside restaurants. He had learned to love *nsima* and goat meat relish and he was sure Vickie would fall in love with his favorite African food, too. However, she said that she was glad for the extra peanut butter and crackers we had sent along -- she just sort of lost her appetite when she learned it was not beef in the hot relish stew! After her shower and shampoo, we took Miss Vickie to her plane in

Blantyre and we doubt those two young people ever saw each other again.

Many times during these early days of meetings with local village leaders and deployment of the door-to-door surveyors, it was necessary to rent two vehicles. One for Ken and one for me. None of the rental vehicles were ever in excellent condition, and only once in a while did we have a car that was in good condition. Since I was my Lord's servant, I trusted him to see me safely at the various destinations. One afternoon I had the privilege of speaking with a group of Christian village leaders about what they could expect to happen as a result of project interventions in the distant and isolated villages. Saying *tsalani bwino* (a form of "goodbye" that actually means "reach your destination well") to these new friends was suddenly interrupted by a plea from one of the women who had walked about 14 kilometers to be at this meeting. She asked, if she and some of her friends might ride a distance toward their village. Of course, I said "Yes!" glad for the company, especially if the old Nissan station wagon should break down. By now, the sun was high and the temperature soaring around 120 degrees Fahrenheit, so I looked forward to the air-conditioned comfort. As people began climbing into the vehicle, they filled up the third seat with five people, then the second seat with another five people, and started to load the front seat with three more! I had to be very firm that only two could ride with me on the front bench seat. Packed in closely, we were off, with the air conditioner turned on HIGH !

However, the only air that entered the station wagon was hot outside air. Nobody at the rental agency told me the air conditioner didn't work! Therefore, we began to roll the windows down just to have movement in the hot air. As I turned the crank on my driver's window, the handle came off and the window fell down into the door! Oh, well, I thought. Then came one of those pot-holed tarmac areas, and try as I did, I couldn't miss them all! Bump! Bump! In addition, the center seat holding five somehow broke and the back fell down onto the feet of the five passengers in the third seat. At the same time, the tailgate door fell off its hinges and just barely hung there. By then, we all were laughing so hard I could hardly drive. Dust boiled up and into those open windows and the rear door. I stopped to inspect and determine what to do and found that one hinge on that back door had been missing and instead the door had been held onto the body with bailing wire. Therefore, I wired it up again as well as I could and in just a few more kilometers, I delivered my laughing passengers to the road that would shortly take them to their villages.

All I wanted to do was keep that poor old Nissan running the rest of the way up the escarpment and into Blantyre and our apartment parking lot! I was weary from the expected wear and tear of the day. I was hungry, and filthy with the dust of the valley caked on my skin and saturating my clothing. I thought of Ken and hoped he was not worried about me being a bit later than we had estimated. Moreover, I made it! I leaped away from what looked like a refugee from the demolition derby and climbed those stairs to the flat. There was no light in the stairway or foyer, and of course, that 6:00 PM African darkness had settled in. No light shone from our windows and I could not see Ken's rental vehicle anywhere. The worst part was that I could not find my key to the flat. Somehow, I was too tired to go for help. I knew that Ken must be coming along soon. Therefore, I lay down and slept soundly on the Welcome Mat until Ken arrived about 4 hours later!

Ken almost tripped on my body as he came into the dark foyer and a shudder of fear turned to relief when I awakened and we shared the stories of the day. Well, we shared the stories after I had a long, luxurious shower! Ken had been working on a village well 'way south of where I had been meeting, and since my vehicle was already gone when he headed for home, he decided he would stop by the Training Center in Ngabu just a little further north. This was the last day of training for the Household Surveyors, and he wanted to be sure their transportation had arrived to take them to their home villages. At the Ngabu junction, he noticed a broken down bus and asked the driver what happened only to learn that this was the bus we had chartered and it was not going anywhere. Its drive line had completely fallen out! Ken found fifty anxious women, ready and waiting, but he told them they would have to wait until he made other arrangements. Fortunately, we had made acquaintance with a professional transporter and Ken was able to contact him and talk him into a late afternoon and all evening task. Ken stayed to encourage the women until they were safely on their way. Time and time again, I felt a little thrill that this practical, patient, and kind man was there with me in Malawi.

The formal training of the HSAs began just one week after the completion of the Door-to-Door Disaster. There was an active Dorika organization at the Ngabu Makande S.D.A. Church. When I asked the pastor to recommend two Dorika leaders who could speak English to help me in planning for the menus for the first wave of training -- the fifty volunteers at a time, for one week -- Rhoda and Jessie stepped forward again! These women knew the government home economist based at the Training Center and with the help of all three we planned the menus, purchased the food and toiletry supplies to keep the trainees happy.

Rhoda took the lead in giving hospitality to the men and women of the bush who made up our trainees. She was there when the buses arrived. She came every morning at wake-up time and conducted morning worship services with them. She checked on special needs and reported them to me so the two of us could decide what to do. However, the most delightful thing Rhoda did was to invite all of the Ngabu Dorika women to come to a Wednesday evening supper and sing-along with the HSA trainees. Rhoda and Jessie served the men and women, however the men in the training class selected their own spiritual leader.Rhoda and Jessie, in their faithfulness to their tasks, taught me so much about unconditional love and hospitality for the bush people. They showed their unselfishness by just being with people they had never seen before. In order to learn their needs, and to serve them; they taught me about bush people food preferences, and where to buy it locally for less than it would cost in the supermarkets of Blantyre. They modeled loving kindness, cleanliness, timeliness, thankfulness and a joyful, worshipful attitude.

All of the curriculum for training the HSAs met and went beyond the government curriculum for HSAs, and it was required by the government that such courses be taught in English. Dutch Dr. Peter taught the physiology of the disease process. Ruth Mkaya, a Registered Community Health Nurse, taught Nutrition, and Management of Diarrhea, the Prevention and Treatment of Parasitic Diseases, Communicable Disease Control, and Immunization Theory and Practicum. The District HI taught Sanitation, Clean Water Development, and Epidemiology. The Director of the Leprosy Clinic, Medical Assistant, Percival Katumbi, taught Leprosy Case Finding and Management of the disease; Nurse Specialist, Grace Chikweza, from Trinity Hospital taught Maternal and Child Health, Family Planning, Village Obstetrics and Midwifery.

These faculty people were paid well by the project. Some of them served on CSAC, and they truly expected to see these HSAs at work in the villages soon. They took great care to teach them well. The HSA students seemed to enjoy the classes and we began to see some positive behavior changes with them. As they learned more about causes of disease, they generally committed to a healthier lifestyle, especially in general cleanliness and dietary elements.

Every day we heard the students singing when it was time for class to begin. They sang religious songs, sad or happy traditional songs, and often broke into dancing until one of their HI supervisors called them to order. Then one of the students would offer a prayer for the day. They lived in the dormitories and all their meals were prepared for them by our well-paid cooks.

At the halfway point in their nine-week training, the HIs suggested in our weekly supervisors' meeting, that we have a celebration, something like an "agape feast." I agreed and they said they would be entirely responsible for the planning. After the date and time was announced, they told all the students and me to bring a special light lunch to exchange with the person whose name we would draw; the two would then eat each other's light lunch together and get better acquainted. What a delightful idea, I thought, and set about planning to bring food items that the natives don't usually have, but often covet, like a chunk of good cheese, cookies, and a bottle of soda pop.

When the time came and we were all seated in a wide circle with Ken included, the HI who served as master of ceremonies, enjoyed announcing a name, then having that person draw another name, announce it, calling for their partner to join them in the center of the circle. The two must then show the group what is in both containers (baskets or plastic bags), ooh, and ahh over it and then find a place to eat together. Suddenly my name was called by the person drawing it from the box. I joined HI, Rex Mauluka, in the center of the room. I curtsied. He bowed and asked me what gifts I had brought him. Therefore, I proudly showed him the delightful and ample light lunch I had with me. Then I asked, "What are the gifts you have for me?" There was dead silence in the room. All eyes were on the two of us in the center. Rex held up for all to see, a light green, grease-soaked paper bag from which he slowly (grinning all the time) withdrew a strange substance. My face revealed the question I did not speak: "What is that?" Rex said, "Take it just as I am holding it. You will love it!" As the greasy object was transferred from his thumb and forefinger to mine, I could see that I was holding a deep fried, defeathered whole bird upside down by its legs. It was so repulsive to me that I felt a wave of nausea, but thinking about this scene in my mind and gulping back the nausea, I took a deep breath and realized that this was a joke on me and that these silent, grinning, staring students and their instructors expected an Izungu performance! Therefore, I gave them one. Wrinkling my nose in disdain, I held the bird up to the light, feigning stomach sickness. I slowly turned around pretending that I would at any minute pop it into my mouth, but gagged and noisily cleared my throat with each move. After several minutes of this agony for me and delighted laughter from my jokers, I was rescued by the District HI who immediately put the whole bird into his mouth, crunching the bones audibly and obviously popping its gastrointestinal tract as he did a little dance, munching and crunching and licking his lips!

Rex then explained to me that these are called "whole chickens" but are actually mature "wagtail" birds are everywhere and easily caught. The "whole chicken" is a delicacy to these people and they are sold in the markets and along the roadsides every day.

Christmas 1991 at Home in Ngabu

We had been in the house on Saopa Road for a few weeks, and by comparison, to the Resthouses where we had stayed, it was heaven! Finally, we were able to use our own personal equipment that we had brought from the US. The queen size bed in an air-conditioned bedroom was perhaps the most appreciated. With the louvered windows throughout this house designed to catch the valley breezes, (to say nothing of scooping in all the red dust from the busy road) it was impossible to cool the entire house. However, Ken is very gifted with general and electrical engineering skills that enabled him to install the air conditioner in the East bedroom window adequately enclosed to cool this one room. We found a custom maker of mosquito netting from whom we purchased a good bed-net. We dipped it in the experimental pyrethrum mosquito-lethal solution (yet harmless to humans) and the most comfortable bedroom in all of Malawi (I thought) was ready. Our choleric personalities keep both Ken and me doing the tasks set before us, making others' work more pleasant and rewarding, and always creating the strategic pathway to achieve our goals. With work styles like this we both needed a good night's sleep, and until we were in our own home in a location that is quiet with cool air, and mosquito protection, we were nearly always in sleep deficit.

The tiny kitchen was adequately equipped with an electric range and refrigerator and a small sink with hot and cold water. The two bathrooms were fully modern and Ken installed our American stack-mate washer and dryer with its necessary electrical transformer in one of the bathrooms. After eleven months in Malawi, we were finally settled quite comfortably in the lower Shire River Valley with the project well under way.

With Christmas coming soon, we were in the mood to celebrate our Lord's birthday with hospitality and a festive function at our home. The Child Survival staff had been deployed to their individual service sites for about three months, so it was also time to bring them in to the Ngabu headquarters for reports, continuing education and affirmations and evaluations. It was a great time to plan a Christmas celebration.

In this poorest of the poor area, little attention is paid to Christmas, except to acknowledge the Holy Birth as the entrance of the Savior of the world. For these Christian people who had nothing of this earth's material goods, except for what the project had provided for them, we felt even the simplest of "Christmas Parties" would be an unforgettable experience. Invitations were sent to all the staff, local government people who had assisted in the project, and to the leaders of the local churches who had been so supportive.

We received warnings that jealousy in the neighborhood might cause some of the people to try to join the party, so we stationed our regular watchman at the chain-link gate to the driveway. He was elegant with an authoritative stance in his new ADRA-provided uniform, and since he was well known and liked throughout Ngabu, there were no gatecrashers.

We lit the walkway to the door of the house with luminaries made of candles in paper bags of sand. Candles also illuminated the entry table and the long serving table in the dining room. Electric lights blazed throughout the house while wonderful sounds of Christmas songs from our good old Emerson radio/cassette player wafted through the opened louvers to the thatched-roof village homes of the neighborhood.

The guests began to arrive with curious, astonished eyes and almost speechless amazement because so many had never been part of a real mealtime celebration for Christmas. I had found a few red and green tinsel-garlands to hang across the archway between the *khonde* (sun-porch entry) and the living room. There was no Christmas tree, no holly or mistletoe, or even artificial boughs to enhance the atmosphere, but the spirit of Christmas was felt by all -- beginning with ourselves.

Our guests had never seen a table set with a punch bowl, glass cups (borrowed from friends in Blantyre) and they had never seen or tasted chips and dips and other American-style appetizers. Ken was concerned when he found two of the HSA women crouched in a corner weeping. When he asked them why they were crying, they responded,

"We are just so happy to be in your home. We have never been invited into an *izungu* home. We are just soooo happy!"

Before the main buffet meal was served, we took time to personally greet all the staff and other guests individually. We sat together, with most of the HSAs on the cement floor, and went around the room expressing gratitude to God for his Son who gives us this kind of love for one another. Some of our leaders from the community were Muslims, but they were most gracious, as they see their Allah-God much the same as our Creator-God, even though most of them did not believe in Jesus as their Savior. The warmth of friendship was almost palpable in that house that night, and the glow of candles added to the sense of loving relationships being shared.

We refrained from inflicting total culture shock in the menu by offering them one of their favorite staples, although not their <u>most favorite</u> food (*nsima*). We served steamed rice with spicy beans and cabbage salad. There was ample French bread from our favorite Portuguese bakery in Limbe, near Blantyre. For dessert, we made an old-fashioned American Oatmeal Cake with coconut topping. They loved the food and ate so heartily that we had to cook an extra pot of rice!

There was only one complaint, and that was in the form of a teasing whine by Mr. McGreen Chideu, one of the HSAs who is the son of Chief Chideu. Mr. Chideu cried loudly that he could not live until the morning without *nsima*. "*Nsima* is the only thing that will satisfy this aching, empty stomach!" -- as he patted a very full belly! Everyone laughed at him, but that was his parting cry as he walked out of our yard, down the dark trail to his quarters.

As our guests were leaving, there came a loud knocking at the back door to the kitchen. Here was a child, bowing deeply and holding a fat, black, live chicken as a gift to us from his parents in honor of Christmas. We, in turn, bowed to this gentle child, took the chicken, and passed the blessing on to McDonald Ntupa, our faithful watchman who had spent the evening at the gate. McDonald's thatch hut where he lived with his beautiful wife and two babies, was just outside our back gate. They enjoyed the unexpected FEAST the next day!

The Christmas celebration continued the next morning as the HSAs arrived at the ADRA office/classroom for continuing education and their own reports of experiences in their villages. We read the nativity story from the New Testament book of Luke and each HSA received a festively wrapped package containing a Christmas card, a red hard-cover King James English Bible, a loaf of whole wheat bread and a one-liter carton of dark red grape juice. From another supply of bread and grape juice we celebrated our Lord's communion using scripture, song, and the sharing of these emblems of His broken body and spilled blood for us. Each one was very touched that they could take home to their families these gifts with so much meaning. Not one had ever tasted real grape juice before, nor had they eaten whole wheat bread -- and to be able to have enough to share just amazed them in this land where there never seems to be enough of anything. Each one of our group of twenty-four stood in turn to give their testimony to each other, and to us, what it meant to them. To be chosen to learn a better way of life and then to be able to teach that better way, demonstrated to them how this change could make a difference in their lives, and in the lives of their country's people.

Cool, Clear Water for Chideu Village

We felt particularly close to Mr. McGreen Chideu for several reasons. One day when Ken and I were returning him to his home village, we received an urgent report that McGreen's father, Chief Chideu, was lying just barely conscious, with a high fever. *Mayi* Chideu, the most senior wife among several, came quickly to meet me and asked if I would come to the Chief's room in the largest thatched house.

As I hurried from the car, I prayed for wisdom, bent low to enter the small door, and found this sixty-year old village leader lying on a bamboo mat on a raised earth bed, in serious condition. I knelt at his side to do what nursing assessment I could. His pulse was rapid; his breathing shallow; his skin hot, dry and dehydrated; and there was a very strong odor that smelled of acetone. When I asked the first wife through McGreen's interpretation if the Chief had diabetes, nobody seemed to know, except for McGreen who thought his father had never been to a real doctor. I asked the family members if they would like me to pray for the Chief, and they eagerly gave me their permission. I just took a moment, to lay my hands on the man's hand, and as flies buzzed around his face, I asked God in His wisdom to give us time to get this child of His to medical care.

We determined that the family and the village elders wanted the gravely ill man taken to the government hospital about thirty kilometers distant. Ken was pleased to make a pallet in the old Toyota, the family members lifted the Chief into the vehicle. McGreen and his mother (the first wife) accompanied Chief Chideu to St. Matthews Hospital, a reasonably good Catholic facility in Nchalo. Fortunately the diagnosis of diabetes and urgent interventions were made in time, and Chief Chideu lived for several more years. This experience bonded us strongly to McGreen and the people of the entire Chideu Village, forever.

Many Malawians suffer from the affects of undetected diabetes. In fact, the average life span for Malawi males before the AIDS epidemic, was about forty-seven years due to the many killer diseases, such as malaria, pneumonia, tuberculosis, and diabetes. One can only imagine what that life span has dropped to now that it is ten-to-fifteen years into this killer epidemic of AIDS.

It was in Chideu Village where our helpful "angel," Akim Kafukiza, lived with his family. Ken soon learned that this enormous village had a real potable water shortage, and he was constantly reminded of this by both Akim and McGreen. As ADRA encouraged Ken to assess the possibilities for development of shallow wells, Chideu Village became an early focus for well development. With Akim's lead, village men dug through the sandy soil to reach water about twenty feet down. To case the well, Ken devised a method using two 40-gallon plastic drums for fruit syrup that he obtained at little cost from the nation's only soft drink bottling company. By cutting the tops and bottoms off the drums and drilling one-inch holes randomly in the sides, then stacking the prepared drums, one atop the other, casing for the bottom-most sides of the well was made. From the top of the upper drum, handmade bricks were cemented into place to finish the casing, a cement cast lid with pump orifice was put in place, and the pump installed.

In this village as all others where shallow wells were developed, Ken established a clean-water committee; the HSAs taught the reasons and needs for clean water; Ken taught the care and maintenance of the well; and the people participated fully in the development and the sense of ownership of their own well.

At last, the women of Chideu Village could obtain their water just a short walk from their hut! But lo, and behold, the water turned out to be quite salty, so it could only be used for washing and bathing, not for drinking. For a time the villagers resumed walking about four kilometers to the usually dry river bed where they dug holes in the sandy bottom and scooped up drinking water about half a cupful at a time, until they had a seven-gallon bucket full. These full, heavy buckets rested securely on the women's heads as they walked the dusty trail back to their huts. Ultimately, ADRA located and developed another site within this village where non-saline water was plentiful.

During the water development in Chideu Village, another improvement was taking place. Akim and his congregation were tired of holding church services under a tree and they began construction of a beautiful bamboo, mud-brick, and thatch church. With a dirt floor, a dirt podium, and tiny high window openings, this church would seat about 200 people. As Ken and I came and went from the well sites, we congratulated the people on their beautiful work on their house of worship for the Church of God. Akim made it clear that when the church was finished he expected me to speak the Word of God to his people!

No amount of my telling Akim that I was not a preacher convinced him and so one day he called at the Saopa Road house to tell me that he expected me to speak to his congregation on a certain Sunday about three weeks hence. So, I humbly agreed to do so, for I had been praying about this potential. I felt I should teach the people about good health and cleanliness, using simple posters and illustrations.

Akim indicated that we might need to hold the church service outside on the hillside because many people would come. The day before I was to speak to the church people in Chideu, I was suddenly very ill with a hot throat and laryngitis, and totally unable to speak. I sent word to Akim to make other arrangements for a speaker, but it was too late for those people who were walking from as much as fifty kilometers away. Nine hundred people came to Chideu Village to hear the *izungu* woman, but their speaker was Akim, himself. Many had risked their lives in walking through neighboring Mozambique jungle to hear about Jesus. It was not the wild animals of the jungle that jeopardized these people; it was the warring factions and bandits that hid in that part of Mozambique during their 20-year civil war.

In consternation, Akim arrived on my doorstep the next day and quickly learned that "the madam" could not speak.

We rescheduled for the next month. Akim told us the stories of how he had ventured into Mozambique even though that nation was in critical civil war and various factions were often on the rampage, killing and burning entire villages. His visits there were always at night, and the people knew he would be there to pray with them and teach them about Jesus. They were so poor from having been robbed by the bandits that ravaged the area that they often wore animal skins and would walk for hours (after dark) to find Akim's meeting places

As I prayed for the right message to give, the answer was totally different than my earlier impressions. Over and over, the Holy Spirit seemed to say, "Just tell them the story of Jesus." When the day arrived, I felt totally at ease, speaking through my interpreter, Albert, one of the ADRA water developers. The goal of my story of Jesus was to help them see Him and His love for them and that He alone has all power over the evil spirits that harass them and keep them in fear. I told them of how Jesus created them, how mankind failed Him and how He came to live on earth to show us what God is like. I told them of how He healed the sick, and raised them from the dead, casting out the demons. I told them the amazing story of about His death and resurrection that overcame Satan, and all evil. By claiming Jesus Christ as our Savior, our sins will be forgiven, and He will give us the power to keep us from falling. As we believe Him, He will make us more loving and trustworthy in our daily life. That the peace He provides us passes all understanding, and someday soon, He will take us to heaven where He is and where there will be no more hunger, sickness, fear, and dying. No AIDS or malaria. No lame people from polio. It took three hours to tell the story with interpretation. I could see that as they listened they began to understand because of the smiles on their faces. In response to me and the good news, they began to nod their heads and chant. Some brought small cans of rocks to shake for rhythm. Pastor Akim began to lead them in singing "Hallelujah" for the God who loves them and takes away all fear. I could not hold the tears back for the joy that I felt in knowing they had seen a glimpse of Jesus through me. In addition to clean water for drinking and washing, the "Water of Life" had flowed freely that day in Chideu Village.

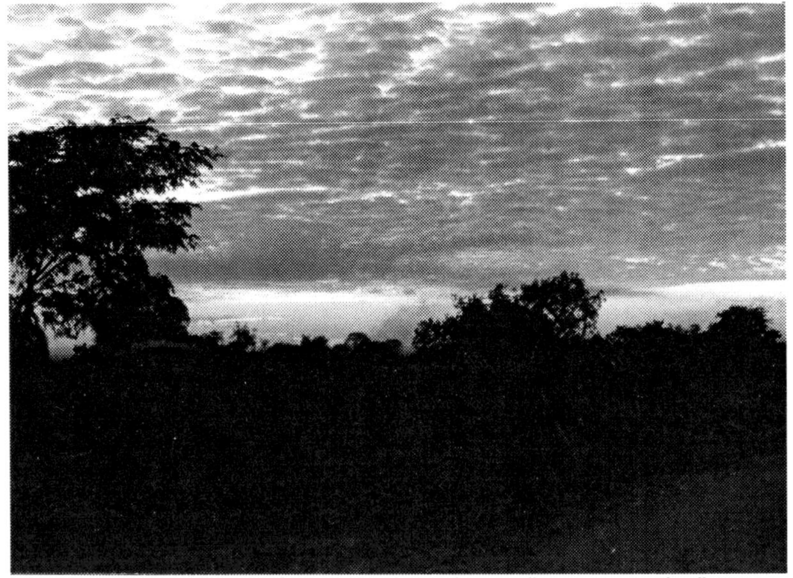

The Sunlight of knowledge clears "moonsmoke"

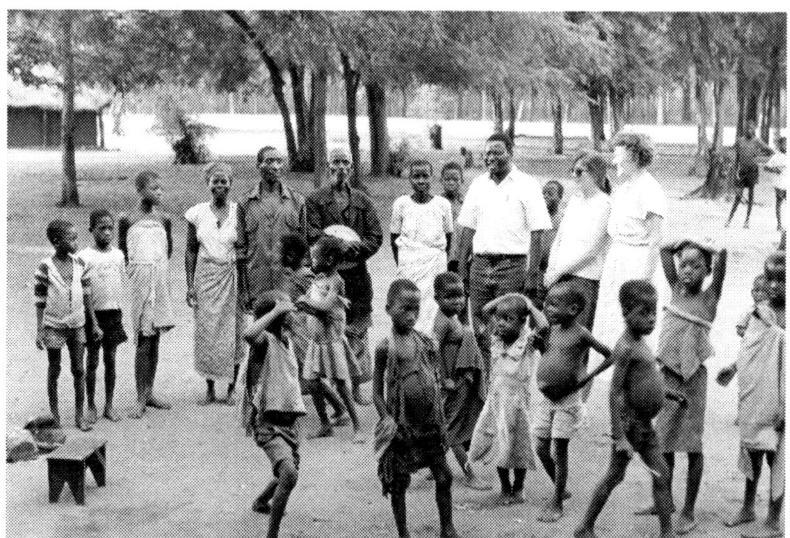

Happy village children...but not healthy

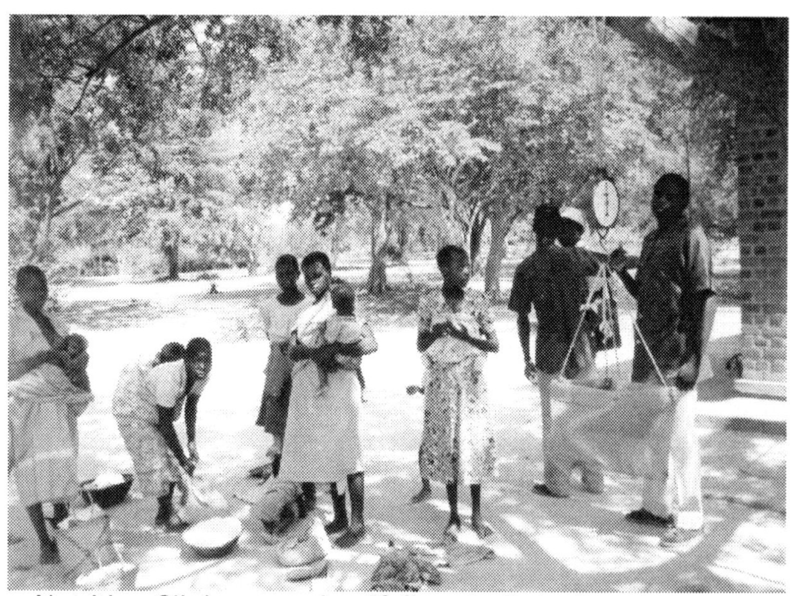

Nutrition Clinic, reversing “failure to thrive”syndrome

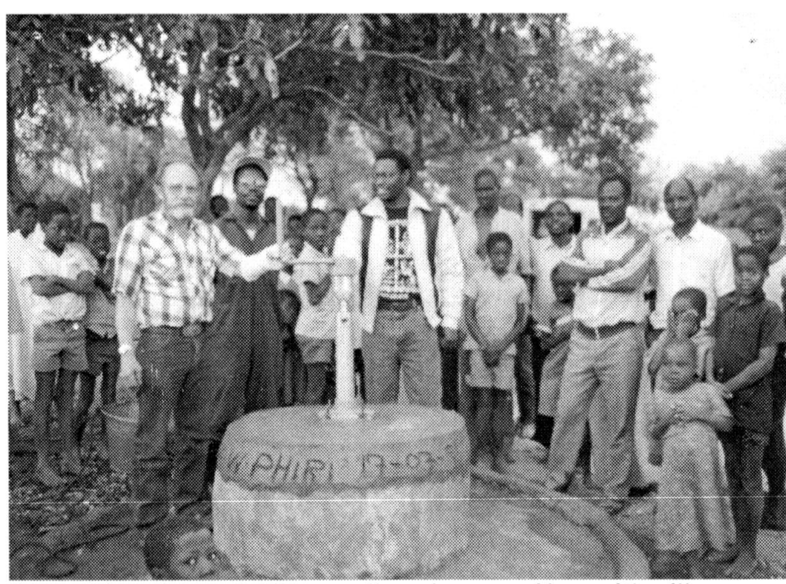

Nyambiru clean,shallow well and pump: Ken with village chief and project Health Inspector...and the children

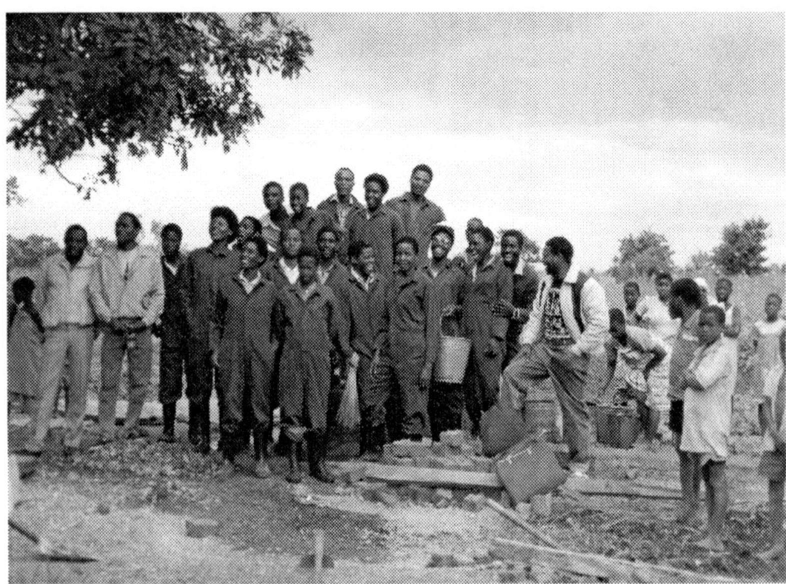

Nyambiru village well: HSAs celebrate completion of their first well

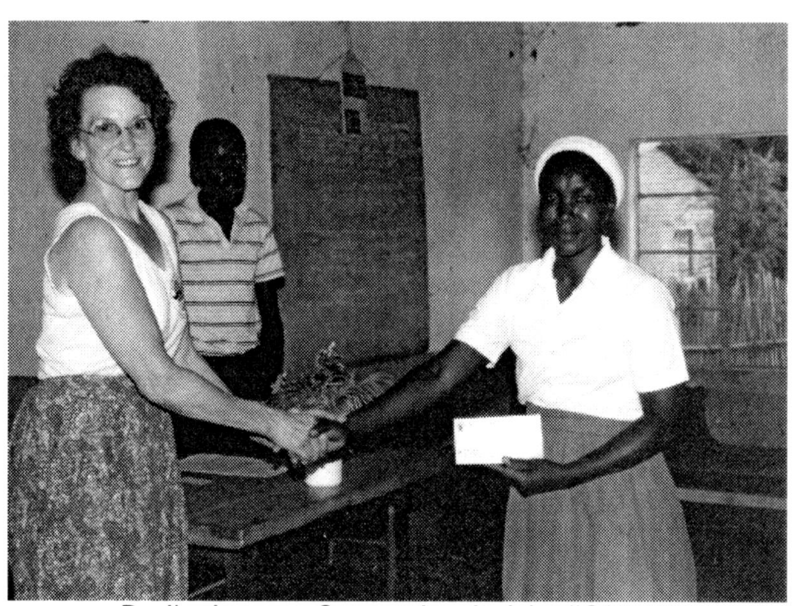
Dorika Income Generation Activity (IGA)
begins with one small check

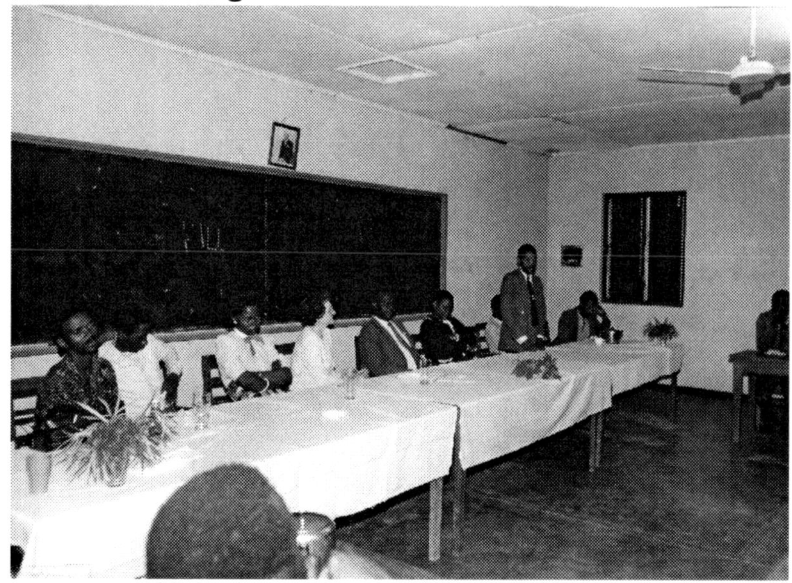
Malawi government officials present
graduation certificates to 22 HSAs.

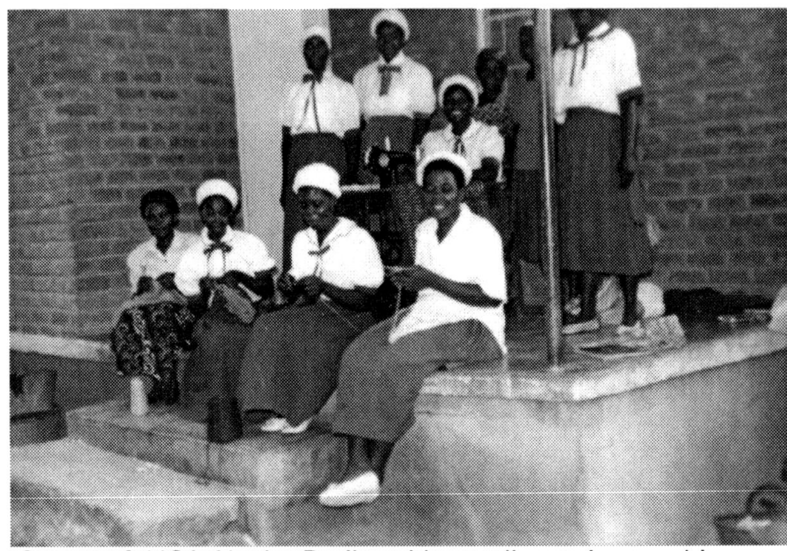

Successful IGA: Ngabu Dorika with treadle sewing machine

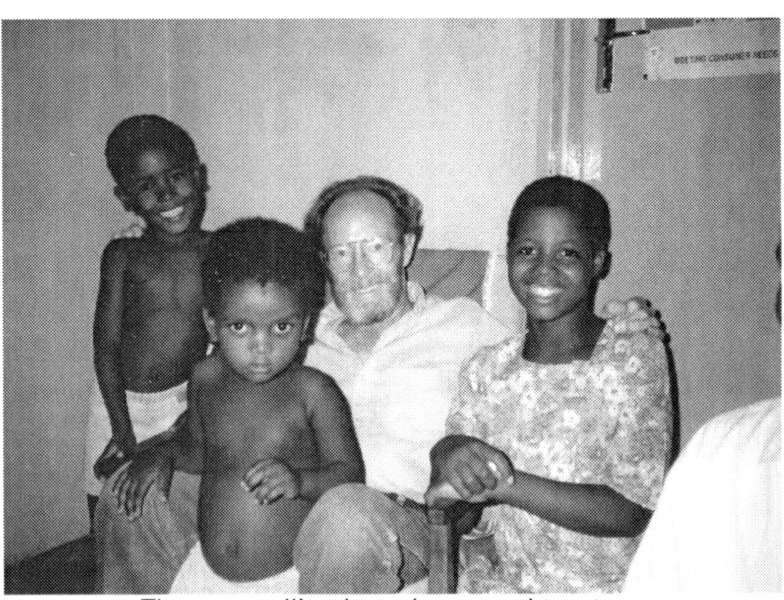

The compelling love, hope and trust
of Malawi's youngest children

CHAPTER 5

Less Moonlight – More Moonsmoke

Difficult Experiences

Even though we were quite sure the selection process had obtained some of the best and brightest student workers in this enormous valley, each one brought his or her own baggage of one sort or another. We had only been under way a few days when we learned that HSA students, Nancy and Jimjones, were husband and wife and that Nancy was pregnant. Well, this was not a cardinal sin, but they had entered the process as single people. So we made nothing of this surprise. But they had another surprise for us. Jimjones was apprehended by the local police who had evidence to prove that he had stolen property from the refugee clinic where he had held a part-time job. So Jimjones was taken to jail in Nsanje *boma* about sixty kilometers south of Ngabu, to serve six months. We felt sad for him and wrote him a letter to encourage him to rethink his life and begin to live an honest life for Jesus and for his family. As a group, we prayed for Jimjones restoration, and Nancy delivered a beautiful baby boy whom she named Jimjones, Junior. Nancy never missed a day of her training or her service and when her husband was released from prison, he found manual labor in Nancy's assigned village and life for this little family settled into normalcy.

Edze – The AIDS Endemic

Pronounce that word as "ed-zee." When our mission to Malawi began, we were told by Malawi health authorities that the Edze epidemic had not yet reached this country except for just a few cases. So we were astonished as we visited Malamulo Adventist Hospital in another section of the bush country, to see dozens of cots in row after row with people in final stages of death lying quietly in many large open-air and screened wards. The Director of Nurses giving us the tour indicated that these dying people were indeed dying from AIDS-related causes, but the government at that time would not allow AIDS to be indicated as the cause. Instead, those in attendance must call the death as due to pneumonia, tuberculosis, or other opportunistic conditions.

About three months into our time there, I received an invitation along with church leaders from every denomination in Malawi to meet with the Minister of Health. The one-day conference was to discuss the possibility of AIDS becoming a major issue in Malawi. Participants would identify and suggest roles for church people and government people to work together to help head off an epidemic like the one raging at that time in Uganda. After introductions and some weak statements from several government health agents, the Minister of Health took charge and put many facts on the table for the very first time. Participants acknowledged that these facts indicated that they had all been asleep as the lifestyles of the people of Malawi had for some time made Malawians easy prey for this devastating disease. It was our privilege that day to write a resolution of partnership among churches and the government to organize and implement AIDS-prevention health education messages to reach every level of the society. A study of the incidence of AIDS in women delivering babies at Queen Elizabeth Hospital in Blantyre showed that 25% of women in childbearing years were either HIV-positive or already AIDS victims. The care of orphans by village relatives and friends became an issue. Demographers could see the nation becoming one populated mainly by grandparents and their orphaned grandchildren.

Shortly after that resolution and admission of the facts, we were thrilled to see ADRA train and deploy several drama teams under the direction of Michael Uzi, professional Medical Assistant and gifted actor. In words and actions, these teams played out powerful dramatizations depicting the real causes, treatments, and deadly finality of this dreaded disease. The teams were in demand by the political party leaders, by local school and University authorities and ultimately by order of the President, every Malawi Army unit received the “Stomp Out AIDS” drama presentations. Michael trained the Child Survival Health Surveillance Assistants in similar dramas and at least three drama teams were developed later by the HSAs for use in all the villages in their locale. Messages included frank reference to how AIDS is transmitted heterosexually after contact with an infected prostitute or drinking partner, then transferred to the several wives. The dramas showed that an agonizing and premature death is the only result for those infected. It was remarkable to see humor woven into the script, even though the subject was so serious.

More and more often the work of teaching in the villages stopped for one week, or two or three weeks, because of the frequent AIDS deaths. Cultural norms required 5 to 7 days of feasting to honor the dead person. Even when food was scarce, villagers would somehow find something for the death festival. Alcoholic beverages brewed from certain jungle plants became very available at these times and often caused other deaths due to toxicity of some of the plants used.

One day I received a letter from the wife of one of the Health Inspectors telling me that it was urgent that she talk with me privately, and soon. I made a special trip to her home in the old Bishop's House at Trinity Parish, about 40 kilometers distant on the East Bank of the Shire River. She told me that her husband had just acknowledged to her that he was HIV-positive and that he has less and less energy to do his work. I had noticed that he often perspired profusely during his times of instructing the class. His wife told me that he spends nearly every night with the prostitutes at the village bar and that she told him she will never sleep with him again because "one of us must stay alive to care for these three children God has given us." This beautiful woman was in great grief as she related her circumstances. I knew that she was a very well educated elementary school teacher and suggested to her that she might need to move back to Blantyre where she possibly could obtain a teaching position. I learned that she had already applied and was accepted to begin teaching at a private Christian school in Blantyre in two weeks. Along with her small teacher's salary, the school would provide modern living quarters for her and her family. Together, we prayed for the future of everyone in her family, including the very ill and misguided father of her children. Then we made an appointment in a few days for Ken and me to transport her children and their entire *katundu* to their new residence at the school. With shame and embarrassment, her very ill husband turned in his Suzuki dirt bike at the Ngabu office, resigned from the project, and caught the evening bus for his parents' home in the far northern part of Malawi.

This Health Inspector had done a very good job in training and organizing the HSAs on the East Bank of the Shire River to continue their work to bring better health to the thousands in their assigned villages. The Lord surely blessed those efforts, and it did not take us long to see a new leader emerge from among the HSAs. Walter Phiri from Bangula-Chiromo had been an acknowledged leader during the nine weeks of training. He had prior health training as an assistant in the Talres Leprosy Clinic at Ngabu and was respected by all his peers. Although we all grieved together at the loss of the Health Inspector and his family, we also praised God together that the work of the project would go on very well with Walter's leadership. In fact, all the HSAs voted to send Walter as the representative from the Nsanje District to the International Conference on Child Survival conducted by the US Agency for International Development that was convened in a Navajo community near Tucson, Arizona. He was very thrilled to have this experience and returned with a wonderful report of comparisons among the various similar projects around the world. In fact, Walter pointed out several lessons he had learned at the conference that would improve our project outcomes.

Only a few weeks after the loss of the first Health Inspector, the other one resigned looking very ill and having lost a great deal of weight. He also had done excellent work while it lasted, though we never heard from him again. By this time, natural leaders had emerged within the group of HSAs so we re-organized the two teams, designating new team leaders and their excellent village health work went on.

CHAPTER 6

STEWARDS OF HIS RESOURCES

Now You See It – Now You Don't

From a project management perspective, one of the greatest concerns I had was accountability for the funds expended to plan and implement the Child Survival work. ADRA was such a new entity in Malawi, without a large budget. Of real concern to me was accurate tracking of the gifts of funds that had been received from the international community of donors and expended in noble services without a real accounting system. I was told not to worry, that in a few weeks we would welcome back to his homeland a young man who was receiving his Master's Degree in Business Administration in the US. This man would serve the Malawi SDA church organization as Assistant Treasurer and he would design the computerized accounting system for all the ADRA programs. These other programs included construction under way for several school buildings, clean water development and gardening projects, besides the Child Survival project with its $500,000.00 three-year budget (the largest of anything under way at that time with ADRA-Malawi).

We were delighted when this new accountant arrived and we turned over our records of expenditures for purchases and payroll. ADRA Directors changed about that time, so both the new Director and I had great expectations for making the entire ADRA-Malawi operation truly business-like. I asked for monthly reports of total expenditures for that month as well as year-to-date records. When I inquired of the accountant why these data had not come to me at the end of his first month he told me that I would have everything I needed the next month.

When no reports were available the second month, the Director, and I decided to see what we could find out together! The Director was anxious, too! The accountant was out of town, so we took this opportunity to look at the file for all of our Child Survival expenditures to date. I recognized all the data that I had submitted in its raw form; I also recognized a receipt for the accountants' new yard fencing at his home, including a dog kennel. Then there were receipts for a "training week-end" away at one of Malawi's lovely resorts. This training had nothing to do with the Child Survival Project. There were at least a dozen other personal expenditure receipts. We asked ourselves why the accountant's personal expenditures were lumped with those of Child Survival.

Since the accountant was supervised by the American treasurer for the church organization, the Director and I took our dilemma to the treasurer. He was astonished and began seeking answers. I assumed that all this would work out, believing that the right authorities now knew of our concerns. In the meantime, the accountant had approval for a business trip to Johannesburg in South Africa, from the Director of the entire church organization for Malawi. We were told that the accountant would return with a much-needed new vehicle for the Child Survival Project. Since we had been awaiting delivery of a vehicle and paying very high rent for inadequate automobiles in the meantime, I was happy to hear the news!

"Well," I thought, "next month I will have the financial information I need to guard the remaining resources of the project." This was one year after we had arrived in Malawi. I was appalled when I learned that this man had experienced a serious vehicle accident that totally destroyed the new pickup truck in the heart of Zimbabwe, about 1200 miles away. Since this new accountant was not injured, he was flying back to Blantyre, leaving the vehicle and the damaged utility trailer full of goods in storage in Harare. We also learned that the wrecked vehicle was not destined for our project, as we had been told!

Many project needs were emerging, the most critical of which was the need to purchase a dependable

vehicle that could carry at least six people and their *katundu* while pulling a loaded utility trailer. Of course, we also needed the utility trailer. We needed adequate electrical transformers for our American-made computers, bedroom air conditioner and the washer and drier. ADRA needed simple water well pumps and other hardware that could not be purchased in Blantyre. After consulting with the ADRA Director, Ken and I decided to fly to Johannesburg where we could purchase the automobile, trailer, and other equipment. We would then return via Harare, Zimbabwe, where the wrecked truck, trailer, and damaged goods were stored. We would take pictures of the wrecked vehicles and bring back all the items that had been salvaged and were in storage. The student HSAs had been deployed and were under capable supervision so it was reasonable to expect the work of Child Survival to continue satisfactorily in our absence. We were off to Johannesburg via Malawi Airlines.

Our dear friends, Ian and Irma Hartley, hosts for our earlier "surgical" visit to Johannesburg were happy to have us stay with them again. They helped us locate all the used car sales lots in the city, which we thoroughly explored without finding any vehicle that met our criteria. However, an ad in the newspaper caught our eye for a 1989 blue Toyota Land Cruiser. We gave it a good trial run, and "Mr. Mechanic" Ken passed positive judgement under the hood, wheels and frame and the deal was made. We completed the transaction at a huge Afrikaaner ranch headquarters. As we entered the office, we could hear a CB radio barking the latest happenings out on the Savannah. There seemed to be uneasiness among the four or five men in the room. The Ranch Manager told us not to mind all the noise, "it is just due to the killings in the townships. We think the blacks are about to begin a mass takeover and we are ready for them! We have our own militia and plenty of ammunition. No matter how they take over, either by government agreement or by revolution, we are ready for them!"

Needless to say, Ken and I were glad to take that blue Toyota and get back to our other purchases! We were aware every moment of civil unrest around us. Radio and TV news reported over ninety people killed in a neighborhood just about two miles from our hosts' home. Even so, it was a bit of a shock to see guards on the roof of the shopping center with their automatic rifles aimed at the parking lot -- they, too, were ready. In downtown Johannesburg, we did a little personal shopping in the most modern of stores. As the hour approached five p.m., the clerks encouraged us to get to our car as quickly as possible. As we walked along toward the car, every shop slammed shut steel bars across the entrances and windows and on every street corner, a soldier appeared with his automatic rifle at ready. We began to appreciate the peace and safety that we had experienced the past year in Malawi and were eager to finish our purchases and be on the way north about 2500 miles through Zimbabwe and Zambia to

Malawi. The shorter route of about 1600 miles was closed at that time due to the civil war in Mozambique.

The rest of the shopping required another day of picking up items we had ordered and loading them into the heavy-duty utility trailer we had purchased. I was driving and made just one wrong turn that took me into one of the black townships that I recognized immediately as unfriendly territory to whites. Glaring eyes met mine from men, women, and children as they peered out of cardboard huts or ran along beside the car. Fortunately, there was a wide spot for me to turn around before very many rocks could hit the car. But my heart was pounding as we got out of there!

We had hoped to leave "Jo-berg" in time to reach Bulawayo, Zimbabwe, for the weekend. We wanted to visit Solusi College there and to see nearby Victoria Falls on our way home to Ngabu. But with too much time spent in Jo-berg and slow going on narrow, pot-holed, black-top roads, we had to forget the lovely side trip and just took a day of rest at Masvingo, capital of Masvingo Province in the heartland of Zimbabwe.

We found a modern motel with a good restaurant and grounds guards who assured us that no one would touch our trailer loaded with goods as long as we left it in their supervision. Just a few miles outside this city lays the great Kyle Reservoir and Game Preserve and the ancient and awesome ruins of the Great Zimbabwe.

The Great Zimbabwe was once a citadel and a holy place. Built between 1000 and 1150 AD, it is constructed entirely of granite building blocks. The Hill Complex comes into view first with its massive curling wall winding around the crest of the hill. Archaeologists have found a treasure trove of artifacts from exciting civilizations that somehow disappeared with what we know had to be disease, drought, and/or overpopulation. We were so entranced that hours just slipped away as we explored these amazing structures.

We still had time to drive slowly through the high grasses

of the Game Preserve where we encountered many varieties of colorful birds, monkeys, baboons and one very large, lazy rhinoceros who just continued his mud wallow, rolling around and over and scarcely looking up at us as we sat safely in the Toyota. Zimbabwe's game preserves are full of a huge variety of animals. We just did not have the time to be in the right place at dawn or at dusk. So we reluctantly left Masvingo and continued our drive to the capitol city, Harare.

As international cities go, Harare just seemed to shine. Bustling modern streets, shopping centers, high-rise financial district buildings impressed us as we drove to the Adventist Divisional headquarters to gain access to the wrecked vehicles left behind the previous month by the Assistant Treasurer. When we found the vehicles, we were truly amazed that ADRA's new accountant, who was also the Malawi Mission's Assistant Treasurer, was not killed with the impact and the rollover. Both the trailer and the truck were just twisted masses of steel. Then we found the storage company and gained release of all the loose items that had been in the truck and trailer. We were a bit surprised to see mostly new personal items that were destined for someone other than the ADRA projects or its people, but we took official control of the items, went a few miles away and bought a strong tarpaulin to cover and tie down our load and continued our trek to the north.

We found a government Resthouse that was clean and engaged a guard to watch our trailer and the vehicle that night. This country was in serious drought at that time and water was scarce, so a real bath or shower was out of the question, but we had enough to drink and to sponge off a bit of the sweat and dust.

About noon the next day, we arrived just outside the Zambia border. We had heard horror stories of the political conditions in Zambia, how police and soldiers are so corrupt that one can never be sure if they are there to keep the peace or disturb it. Zambia and Zimbabwe at that time were both under Communist rule. But where Zambia seemed almost entirely dependent upon "big-mother," the Soviet Union to subsidize the economy, Zimbabwe seemed economically stable and much more like a democratic nation. We were cautious as we approached the border, wondering what to expect. As we came to a British Petroleum service station in a stand of tall eucalyptus trees, we decided to fill up the tank and freshen up with a cold soda. Pop machines are everywhere in Africa, we thought. It was a good thing we enjoyed both the full tank and the cool soda, because there was little petrol and no pop machines in Zambia.

Parked under that eucalyptus tree we were suddenly surrounded by a herd of about a dozen wild elephants! They had just sauntered out of the bush and were curious about our vehicle. They quietly, one-by-one, marched around our rig, sniffing nearly every inch, then raising their trunks in the air. We sat there silently!, barely able to breathe for the excitement of being up so close that we could look right into their mouths, the ends of their trunks and those great, wise eyes. What damage they could do if we should startle them in any way, we thought! Then, suddenly, without any real sound, they shuffled off into the forest again. Whew!

Immigration authorities at this Zambian border were very slow, very gruff and demanded to know all about us. They reviewed our shipping documents for all the materials we carried. While they were doing this laboriously, an 18-wheeler trucker told Ken that he had been there at the border for three days waiting for clearance, and that we might as well just plan to camp there for a few days. We prayed that this would not be so. Indeed, in only about two hours, we were all but finished with processing, when we were directed to drive to a certain point for inspection. This was a Tsetse Fly inspection! A man in a pith helmet with a flashlight and a can of insect spray inspected all the wheel wells and sprayed his insecticide into them, then took his time writing down our vehicle data before waving us off to cross the entire nation toward Malawi! Our worst fears just turned into a comic memory of (tame) wild elephants and Tsetse Fly inspectors!

We were accustomed to the Malawi countryside with its primitive, but vigorous farming efforts. Here in Zambia, most of the farms appeared abandoned. The little roadside towns had no merchandise in their shops; people who lived there all seemed to be beggars at the road's edge. The tarmac road in Zambia was in terrible disrepair with constant surprises of potholes and drop-offs. Wherever we looked, there seemed to have been years of neglect and degradation.

Out in the middle of nowhere we came upon the only village that did not seem to be depressed. It was an area where a soft marble-like stone was just under the surface. We called it "soap-stone," and the native craftspeople were everywhere, urging us to buy their carvings. Ken made his selection and I made mine, and when we got into the car we had both bought similar beautiful stone carvings of a mother with her children! We both had similar impressions as we enjoyed these carvings that spoke to us of the gentleness of motherhood even in those hard times.

Then came Lusaka, the capitol city of Zambia. We were appalled. The streets were filthy with everything from human excrement to torn papers and rags and the blown in dust from the dried up fields. Nearly all of the former shops were closed, or boarded up. Sad-faced people were walking everywhere, but nobody seemed to be going anywhere in particular, they were just walking and staring and sad. It seemed that everyone we saw or met in Zambia was sad in those days.

We needed more fuel and watched for a BP station that would be most likely to have a supply. Shortly we noticed not only a BP station with lights on, but attached to it was a store that had a sign that said "Super Market." We had no idea where we would sleep that night or where we would find food, so I was delighted for what I thought would be a chance to purchase fruit, cookies or crackers and perhaps some cheese or peanut butter. These are common items in Malawi markets. But when I entered this little store, there was nothing on the shelves except a few cans of cooking oil, some maize meal, and beer. No packed nuts or sweets of any kind. No bread, crackers, biscuits, or cookies. No fruit or vegetables. And no cold soda in the cooler, only some locally made beer. We knew that indeed, we were among the poorest of the poor, and besides that, they were sad and dejected as an entire population. So we just drove as far as we could that evening until we found a government Resthouse where the cook had not left for the day! He made us hot, steaming bowls of rice and some kind of meat and curry sauce. It was delicious, for we were really hungry. And I thought, "I believe this is the first time in my life I have experienced real, insatiable hunger! It had been at least twelve hours since we had eaten a few sour oranges. I began to realize some of the reasons for the mass sadness we saw and felt that day, most of these people had not had enough to eat for perhaps months. We slept soundly, again with a government guard on watch over our vehicles.

The next day brought us to the Malawi border and its immigration officials. We were greeted pleasantly, almost as if they had been watching for us! We soon found out why! These immigration officials had received advance notice of our leaving Zimbabwe and estimated day of arrival at the Malawi-Zambia border. The inspector headed straight for that trailer and asked to see our shipping papers from the storage house in Harare. We produced them and he asked us for full information as to how we came to be transporting these items when they had been purchased by an official "for the Seventh-Day Adventist" church, but consisted mostly of toys, soccer balls, soccer shoes in various sizes, a couple of television sets, a VCR, a washing machine and other personal household items. We told him that we honestly had no idea of the purposes of the items, we were just told to pick them up and bring them to church headquarters in Blantyre where the official who purchased them is employed. The inspector conferred with other inspectors and decided to impound a couple of the most expensive items until the official in question and/or other church officials could explain why these items should be duty free. We felt almost guilty for carrying items that were not legitimately duty free, yet were transported in the name of the church. We were embarrassed, but they assured us that they would not be dealing with us -- we were the unwitting transporters. So we left a TV set or two behind.

The next thing we noticed on re-entry to Malawi was the persistent happiness on the faces and attitudes of the people everywhere. As poor as the Malawians are, they rejoice at the least blessing they experience. Although this nation was not yet a democracy, Malawi had never experienced Communism as had spilled out over Zambia from "big mother," the USSR. Individuals and families in Malawi had been allocated land and were expected to till it for food -- enough food to sell or barter, in some cases. A certain type of tribal pride and individual self-worth seemed to prevail. The national slogan spoke of this ethic as brochures reached around the world: "Malawi, the warm heart of Africa." Such a contrast with the sad faces we had just left behind. By contrast, the general "face" of the people throughout Zambia at that time exhibited sadness, which we felt, must have come at the recent end of Communist USSR support and the people simply left the communes where they had learned dependency. They owned no land themselves. Their supply lines and general commerce had broken down, for the land and the national economy remained in the hands of an elite group of corrupt leaders.

Accountability

As we returned to the fully functioning project and that comfortable house on Saopa Road, we thanked God for the richness of the experience of that trip and for His protection along the way. We also thanked Him for keeping our project on track. The project staff and students rejoiced for the blue Toyota and the trailer that would transport them to their workstations and do the many other important tasks in completing our work. That Toyota Land Cruiser and utility trailer would carry the HSAs' *katundu*, haul pumps, cement, and other well building equipment to those villages where Ken and other ADRA people were putting in shallow wells.

It was time for our annual report to USAID, and to ADRA International in Maryland. Once again, I asked the Assistant Treasurer for the financial income and expenditure spread sheet for that full year. What I received made no sense whatsoever. In addition, the payroll was totally askew for the third month in a row for our project's 27 staff.

I wrote that Annual Report and expressed grave concern that the year end expenditures were not accurate, but that we would attempt to give the correct figures within three months. Then I presented a copy of that report to the ADRA Director, to the Treasurer and his Assistant, and to the Director of the Malawi Union Mission of Seventh-day Adventists, in addition to the copies that went to ADRA and USAID offices in the United States. I asked the Treasurer to meet with me and his assistant, whose duty it was to perform accurate fiscal accounting and reporting. My goal was to enter into a problem-solving effort to obtain accurate accounting for the entire project and appropriate payroll management.

When the three of us met, the Assistant Treasurer had no answers for his "funny-figures" in the annual report. He did agree to comply with the necessary procedures for accurate payroll. At this time, I presented the problems to both the ADRA Director and the Director of the Malawi Union Mission, S.D.A. The ADRA Director acknowledged his concern but felt that I needed to express my concerns in person to the Malawi Union Mission Director. I was eager to do this, but something happened that postponed that meeting and landed me in the hospital with a king-size bellyache.

Yes, it was a pyloric ulcer at the outlet of my stomach. And I had never had a stomachache before in my life! Zantac, rest and careful diet the next few days calmed my gut, but also gave me time to formulate my plan for talking with the Mission Director. I asked him that the Assistant Treasurer be taken off the ADRA Child Survival accounting completely, and that ADRA be allowed to hire its own trustworthy accountant. Ken and I had agreed that if this change did not occur within sixty days, we would need to leave the project.

So the leading S.D.A church official in Malawi, the Mission Director called for an external auditor and notified ADRA International that something was wrong. When I received a call from the ADRA office in Maryland, I was told that the situation could not possibly be as serious as I was seeing it. They suggested that Ken and I take a holiday at a nice Malawi resort and we would feel better! When I asked what they thought of the Annual Report, they had to acknowledge that they had not read it. Doesn't anybody care what happens to the tax dollars of my country? Doesn't anybody care that there is no accountability for the dedicated offerings of humble people of the church? Those church offerings made up 25% of the funds for this project! USAID (US taxpayers) provided 75%. The ADRA officials seemed to just want me to keep quiet. So I suggested that if they did not insist on sound accounting practices here in this project, I would make a special report directly to USAID. Quickly, they asked me not to do that and assured me that they would look into the matter.

In a few days an auditor arrived from Harare and after spending about twelve hours going over the Child Survival files, he threw up his hands, telephoned me, and told me that the situation was impossible to audit. He calculated that at least $30,000.00 was totally unaccounted for. I never saw his report to ADRA or to the Malawi Union Mission.

When sixty days had elapsed and we still had no change in accountant or the system, Ken and I gave our 30-day notice to leave the project. Since we were close to the mid-course formal evaluation of project outcomes, we were asked to stay at least until the evaluation was complete. We agreed to do so, and began to search for our replacement Project Manager.

Suddenly, one day the Assistant Treasurer resigned and ADRA recruited its own accountant. Then, and only then, did ADRA International send its accountant with software for a fine computerized accounting system which he installed in ADRA Malawi's computer! We were delighted that our voices had finally been heard and corrective action was under way. To this day, we do not know if that Assistant Treasurer ever had to pay duty on items he had purchased for himself (probably some for resale) with Child Survival money. We do not know whether he was ever held accountable for missing funds, but that is God's business, not ours. Ultimately, in this life and the next, there is accountability.

My stomach ulcer began to heal. But by then, both Ken and I succumbed to Malaria, even with having taken preventive medicine. The illness just knocks the wind out of one's sails for several weeks. The project staff were doing a fine job teaching health and organizing huge villages for clean up and sanitation efforts. We continued to attend the graduation ceremonies as the Village Mother Visitors began their work in teaching the mothers health protection, disease prevention, and management of common illnesses.

You Can't Trust 'Em!

From the first day we arrived in Malawi, we were warned by "seasoned" missionaries about the inability to trust the Malawi people. "They will steal you blind!" we heard frequently. "Keep everything under lock and key; watch your clothes hanging on the line and count every item that your housekeeper puts in the washing machine, so that you can tally every item as you put them away." The warning lists went on and on. "Never trust the Malawi police – just treat them like they are stupid, and they will be confused and not bother you."

These warnings came from experienced Americans who had lived and worked in several parts of Africa. At first, we took them seriously. But as we became acquainted with the police at several government checkpoints, we found they were real people. They seemed to have our best interests at heart as well as their surveillance jobs to do. At the Kamuzu Bridge checkpoint on the way to our Nsanje District, the police came to know us as "The Bible People" after one of them asked us for a Bible and we delivered it. Then they all wanted one, and we were only too happy to present them each with a Bible. Some wanted the Bible in their native language of Chichewa, and others wanted theirs in English. As soon as the International Bible Society people in Blantyre learned that we were "The Bible People," they provided us with Bibles by the case!

Wherever we went, we found that as we treated these dear people with respect, we received their respect. In the valley, where our work was, we never had a single item stolen. Once, in Blantyre, we had a bag full of dirty clothes stolen out of our unlocked vehicle. Where the people knew us, we were entirely safe and very much loved. We have decided that human beings, no matter what race or nationality, need respect, acceptance and love, and where we model those attributes with sincerity, we receive the same attitudes in return.

CHAPTER 7

GOD'S GREATNESS IN OUR WEAKNESS

Cups of Cold Water

Water – cool, clear water is always a human survival issue in sub-Sahara Africa. Malawi, with its great-rift valley, rivers and streams must depend upon the unpredictable rains for growing their crops and for daily human consumption. The Malawi government, with help from various donor nations, had attempted to establish a system of wells and pumps to serve villages within short walking distance. What we found in the huge Nsanje District were broken pumps and dry well holes, except for a few still functioning, hand-cranked, pumps. Many villagers were miles away from fresh water supply, necessitating the women of the village to walk two or more hours to and from their homes, to carry five to seven gallons home on their heads. Other villagers boiled the river water (when there was water in their river) or used the three-pot method of purification of water from shallow, dry, riverbed holes.

Improving the water supply was a priority expressed in our Detailed Implementation Plan. Ken quickly picked up on what his role might be in implementing a village-by-village assessment of water issues and the village leaders' interest in improving the availability of potable water in close proximity to their homes. Ken found eleven villages (approximately 30,000 people) in dire need of water! Funds were available for hand-turned pumps, casing materials and transport of these materials to well sites. With the mighty Shire River flowing year around, through our project region, the underground water table was about twenty feet down through sandy soil. Before making any promises to the village leaders, Ken insisted that they appoint a "Clean Water Committee" to help guide the project. The committee, usually members of the "Village Health Committee" that the HSAs organized, would arrange for workmen, decide on the location of the well, learn the workings of the pump and set up a maintenance plan to repair pumps as needed in the future. This responsibility in the hands of the village people was a kind of "first" for them, because all the old, failed wells were government controlled, and villagers were told to leave them alone if the pumps broke or there were any other troubles. As Ken and his helpers inspected government wells that had not been used for several years, he learned that the pumps were simply worn out. In meeting with the government "water officials" he learned that there was never any budget to repair or replace pumps. The Clean Water Committees assumed village ownership of the well and all water uses and the necessary future improvements and maintenance. These were their own wells! And they loved working with Bambo Ken. Oh, they wanted to call him, "Master" as they had been taught to do with government leaders. But Ken would have none of that and insisted they call him "brother." They would not let him lift a shovel or mix the cement...all manual labor was their job! And they ultimately came to call us "father and mother."

Although these were shallow wells in every case, they required casing and protection at the top which was about 3 feet in diameter for 15 to 30 feet down. Ken was able to procure fruit syrup barrels for all the shallow wells that connected at the top to a cement platform and cement cover especially designed to conform to the pump in final installation.

No well was installed without the guidance of the local Ministry of Health representative who was usually a qualified Village Health Inspector. They knew the history of the locale; the logical terrain for a successful hand dug shallow well, and the water habits of the local villagers. We made "Clean Water Development" a major part of the training of our HSAs and involved the District Ministry of Health HI as their instructor. To pass the course, each trainee needed to pass a written examination and participate in every aspect of development of at least one successful shallow well. In preparation for this practical experience, the project provided coveralls for the entire class and "gum-boots" as they called the black rubber boots that were produced from Malawi's one rubber plantation.

The Nyambiru Clean Water Experience

The project students' demonstration well was chosen to be located in a village where there was high, endemic, incidence of cholera that was directly traced to contaminated drinking water. The village was very poor in that it was located over ten kilometers from the Shire River, and drought nearly always took their crops of maize, groundnuts, cotton and guar beans. They had very little to sell or to trade for their subsistence food. But this was their home for past generations, and when it did rain, they shunted water to a pond and in ignorance, saw this pond as clean water because it came from the rain. However, their pigs, goats, chickens, and cows frequented this pond also as their best water supply. In the many dry years, the pond completely dried up and cattle were driven several miles to another pond. There had never been a government well installed within the 10-kilometer radius of the village.

With the help of Rex and James, the project Health Inspectors, Ken set about educating the villagers about the need to dig a good well for good water so that many deaths would be avoided. Once the site for the well was determined, and the Clean Water Committee appointed by the village chief, the village was persuaded to fence a wide area that would surround the well to keep the animal feces far from the surrounding sandy soil. The women in the village were excited to learn that the well would also provide a cemented chute for water to reach a waist high cement-washing table." Clean clothing would replace the smelly rags they wore until they could get to the other pond, or even further to the big river to do laundry! The Child Survival Project HSAs turned the first shovel of soil to begin the dig, but the villagers took over as they were guided by our students. In less than a week, the SoBo beverage syrup barrel casing was installed and clean water was pooling about 20 feet down!

The day that the cement cover and cement-washing table were finished and the pump was to be installed was a day of celebration for the entire village, our project trainees, and their supervisors, and certainly for Ken and me. As the first cool, clear water gushed from the pump turned by one of the student leaders, shouts went up from several hundred people gathered around! There was high-pitched ululating from some of the women, and the traditional dancing celebration began. Cups of cold water were passed around and the HSAs began a song of gratitude to God for His supply of *madze odzidzirwa.* It is a moment we will never forget, being a part of so much joy and gratitude. Yes, we all danced with the villagers to share our joy. Then, the village chief invited all of us to stay and eat a festive meal they had prepared. The chief's deep voice rumbled across the village as he lifted his hands to thank God for the work of the HSAs and this wonderful miracle of clean water for their village. After washing hands in the stream of clear water from the new pump, we sat around the common pot on bamboo mats on the ground under a tree. We felt our spirits bonding with these precious people as they took one more step toward health. From the common pots on our mat, we ate with our fingers, *nsima* dipped in relish, a hot sauce made from okra and goat meat, seasoned with salt and a chili spice.

Far Away Places

One day, leaving the students under the direction of HI Rex Mauluka and their instructors, James and I took the old blue Toyota to visit the two farthest outposts in Malawi, Misamvu and Kanyimbi villages. We went South on broken tarmac to Bangula; then West, fording a river and up through the forest of ebony trees where baboons peered at us and scampered out of the way. Higher and higher, we climbed. There really was no road, just a wide footpath. Stopping at the gate to Mavdbe Game Preserve, we were met by the game warden with his big smile, asking for our credentials and the purpose of our visit. He recognized James because only a few days earlier, James and Rex had taken their Suzuki's up this trail to investigate the interest of the village leaders in having a qualified health worker come to them. With the game warden's permission, we continued through the game park, seeing many impala, the tiny Suni deer, ornery warthogs, a few curious monkeys, and many screeching and scrambling baboons, trying to keep up with us while warning us to stay out of their forest. The terrain became more and more rugged with an occasional boulder to stop for and push or roll out of the way. Seventy kilometers away from the valley, we came to Misamvu. The chief, headman, and MCP leader met us under the trees and brought me a small wooden bench to sit on.

James was a good interpreter, and we went over our proposal again with them. We would set up an HSA to live in their village, help them with their illnesses, and teach them how to be healthier, especially dealing with the mothers and children under the age of three. The village would need to provide a house and agree to establish a health committee to work with the HSA. With tears of joy in their eyes, and big, nearly toothless smiles, they assured us that they would provide the "best house in our village" and took us there to see a fine little brick home that had been built for a primary school teacher, but the government never sent the teacher. "We have been praying for a health doctor and now you are bringing us someone. You are an answer to our prayers," they said. Although very remote, we knew this was the right thing to do, and gave them the approximate date they could expect to see the blue Toyota again bringing their resident HSA.

On the return drive, I asked James if he could stay in a place like Misamvu. There obviously was no general market for goods or services; no itinerant merchant brought goods in a vehicle over that trail. Local people bartered with one another for foodstuffs and once in awhile the hardiest of them made the long journey afoot to sell a chicken or goat in order to buy clothing or medicine.

James indicated he was not sure he would be willing to stay very long. I thought about what it would take for me to do it, and the thought came that if I could go home to the valley once in awhile, I could do it. So I suggested to James that perhaps we should tell the HSA who volunteers for this large, remote village, we would bring him/her out to their home village every other week end, -- home on Friday and returned early Monday. James thought that would be a very good plan, and so it was decided.

We took the fork in the road that took us thirty kilometers out to Kanyimbi where we had an almost identical experience as that at Misamvu, and once again, the HSA would live in an unused teacher's house. They told us that they had only had this elementary school for five years, and they had been praying for a clinic. "Will your health man bring medicine? We need medicine when we get sick." "Better than medicine, the health man brings himself to teach how to stay well, to help you treat common problems and to organize your people to help each other", I responded.

At that time we were negotiating with the pharmacy division of the Ministry of Health to purchase a few simple medicines such as the Quinine preparation for Malaria (in use at that time), Aspirin and the anti-diarrheal salt-sugar preparation for oral rehydration liquid for infants and children's diarrhea, and Vitamin A. We had discovered that a thin soup made from only the liquid of steamed rice or maize seemed to give better healing results for the tiny babies suffering from diarrhea than the WHO standard salt-sugar preparation. But we were not yet ready to talk about medicines with these villagers, except for the immunization materials, which we had obtained from the District Health Officer.

James and I felt very satisfied that our people would be welcome in these villages and perhaps we could show the Ministry of Health how it could be done. The District Health Officer had told us it would be nearly impossible for anyone to serve these villages due to the distances and lack of roads, goods and a market.

One of the criteria for acceptance into the training was that individual HSAs must be willing to move from the comforts of their own village to one of the distant needy places where no health worker had ever been. Of course, these finalists had said they would be willing to move, but I wondered how it would be when we came right down to the deployment and that move. So a few weeks before the course was completed, I placed maps of the valley on the walls of our office, indicating the neediest villages with colored pins. Malawians seem to have difficulty-understanding distance and space, so interpreting the maps was a most difficult exercise for them. I colored the river blue and wrote "East Bank" and "West Bank" and showed them that the colored pins really represented the villages where none of them lived. There were thirteen of the HSAs who already lived in target, high-risk villages. With the guidance of the District Health Officer, we identified eleven villages that were neglected. Therefore, we had eleven colored pins. The HSAs finally caught on that eleven of them would need to move.

I suggested that they needed to think what a move would mean to them. Maybe it would be just one great adventure, being a missionary to their own people. Or perhaps they had always wanted to live someplace else. Or maybe they had a friend or relative who lived in one of those distant villages and it might be nice to be near them. I asked them to think of all the reasons they might like to be on the front line, helping their nation to develop as they helped families to achieve a better way of life in order to save some of the children from dying unnecessarily. I told them that three days before their graduation exercise, I would ask them to write down their first, second and third choices of villages to serve and give their written choices to the HI who would be supervising that area east or west of the river. I did not hear much talk about this subject, but felt sure there was much heart searching and a lot of dormitory talking after hours.

The day came for their written decision, and ten HSAs had made clear choices. Only one had a difficult time because she was having family problems at home.

Elizabeth's husband worked in Blantyre, living with one of his other wives there, while she was expected to raise their three children in her village. She was surrounded by alcoholic relatives, none of whom were safe to help her with the children. So we worked with her and made a special deployment locale for her so she could care for her own children. I was amazed at what God had done in the hearts of these dear student HSAs, to keep them committed to serving their people in nearly forgotten places. As they received their village assignments, nearly all of them achieved their first choice, so none were really disappointed. The reasons for their choices were as many as there were HSAs: curiosity, mystery, they'd never been there, a relative already lived there, etc.

After graduation day, the HSAs would have one week or two off with pay to get ready for service in their own assigned high-risk village and others to get their *katundu* ready for Ken to transport them to their posts. I praised God that the decisions for deployment had been made so well by these precious people.

Celebrating Progress

Every morning, as we convened the HSA class, there was spontaneous singing and often, dancing. Many of the songs were well known hymns that I easily recognized, but sung in Chichewa. With hands clapping and bodies moving, and a wide range of harmony merging in chorus, the students sang from their hearts. Sometimes the songs would go on to joyful, traditional songs of plenty, of love, marriage, and fertility! Usually the traditional songs called for the accompanying dance, and they would have gone on for hours had not the supervisors called them to order.

Whatever doubts or concerns I had in my mind as I came to the classroom from home, I was always lifted and encouraged by the sounds of singing. One governmental official commented that he had never heard so much singing from any group before, and he wanted to know if I had recruited only the gifted singers! I assured him that we had recruited dedicated people who could lead and teach their people, and God threw in the musicians!

Each day when class was called to order, they would stand while one member of their group offered a prayer for God's guidance for the day. Sometimes, they would insist on teaching me the words of their songs. Their language is fairly easy to learn, since it is strictly pronounced, phonetically. One little song that we sang together often is known in English as *God is So Good.* The Chichewa words are:

Mulungu wabwino, Mulungu wabwino,
Mulungu wabwino, abwino, gy ine.

(God is so good, God is so good,
God is so good, He's so good to me.)

Conversely, it was fun for me to teach the students some of our American songs, such as, *There's A Sweet, Sweet Spirit In This Place,* and they thoroughly enjoyed singing and playing some American children's games like *The Hokey Pokey* and *London Bridge is Falling*!

Revolt in the Troops

It was time for the quarterly week-end workshop for the staff. We tried to plan something for everyone: the office secretary, the cleaning lady, the Horticulture team, the HIs and their teams of HSAs. We heard their reports, problems and pleasures; they heard the latest news from ADRA and the Child Survival Program; we read scripture, inspirational stories, sang songs, did dramas and dances; we did problem solving and always had one day of health principles education. The program paid for their bus fare from their station back to Ngabu, except for the two who worked far beyond the end of the bus line. Ken drove out there and brought them into the office classroom. For those whose homes were away from Ngabu area, we arranged for their rooms and food allowances.

One morning, tall and elegant Mercy Njiragoma entered the office-classroom in a slouched position and sat down hard on the bench with eyes lowered and with a big sigh. Honex Faind Phiri had a similar downcast attitude that was visible, and when usually vivacious Jessie came in she sat near the other two. The rest of the staff entered and took their places. Before their teammate could begin his worship talk and have prayer, Mercy asked if she could speak.

Giving her permission to speak, I wondered what was coming. She and her two sad allies had decided that some unequal treatment was going on, and they believed that for the three of them who had homes there in Ngabu it was not fair that they did not receive the same food and lodging stipend as those whose homes were elsewhere. Then Mr. Honex Phaind Phiri rose, asking to speak, and again laid out the same scenario, although more forcefully. Then Jessie Kadzibwa, with angry eyes flashing announced still more forcefully, that the three of them would resign unless they received the same allowances that the others received. Through this sudden and surprising eruption, I was silently praying for wisdom as how to respond. As their manager, I guarded our resources and tried to apply equality measures everywhere. I felt the Holy Spirit guiding me, for I had no right answers, and just waited for His leading. After a moment of silence and with my gaze steadily upon Mercy, Honex and Jessie, I felt mental energy enough to say that they could be excused from that day's activities and that I would meet with the three of them the next morning. They stomped angrily out of the room, stopped outside to confer with one another before heading off in their separate directions.

I couldn't sleep much that night and prayed for direction. By morning it seemed clear that a compromise was in order. They clearly were not entitled to the sleeping room stipend, however I began to see that no food allowance could be considered an inequity as they often arrived in their homes there in Ngabu that might be bare of foodstuffs. So I had a proposal in mind when the three of them arrived, quite late, at the appointed place. I opened our discussion with a brief prayer and shared that in the night I realized that part of their complaint needed attention. Then I indicated that my prayerful decision was that they each would receive food allowances while staying in their own homes, but no housing allowance. I expressed to them how treasured they were to the project – God's work for their own people; and that they would be a great loss to their people if they should resign. They were silent and sad faced at my proposal and asked to leave to confer with one another. After a few minutes they returned and said that they needed to hold to their original demand. If it was not met, they would resign and report me and the project to the government Ministry of Labor that, they informed me, "puts people in jail forever" for any uneven or unfair treatment of employees. I told them that they could not return to their posts or the workshop with that attitude, and that I believed that even the government authorities would see my compromise offer as fair. I prayed aloud with them and gave them three days to accept or be terminated.

Honex and Jessie were in class that day, sober but surrendered! At the end of the third day, Mercy slowly entered the class-room, rolling those big black eyes at me and giving a sidelong grin. By then all the staff had heard something of the ultimatums exchanged, and they all stood and applauded Mercy's return to the group. After class they all received their food allowance and returned to their usual enthusiastic, hard-working HSA styles.

There is something in their culture that makes these

lovable people very competitive and always "keeping score". I often noticed that they watched to see if I spent a little more time with one of them and would invent ways (either as a group or singly) to divert my attention from one to the group or to one of them who had a singular need. They vied with one another to spend time with *Bambo* Ken as he transported them between Ngabu and their village posts. They kept track of us in so many ways. Ken and I did not find it difficult to accept such scrutiny, since they all had so many needs and we loved them individually as well as the group

Graduation

When we lost two of the talented trainees to their own choices and resignations, we grieved deeply. However there were twenty-two wonderful reasons with whom to celebrate their nine weeks of training. Every one of them had endured the training, testing and demonstrating newly acquired knowledge, skills and abilities. Those experiences had changed their lives immensely. The first resignation came early in the program when one of the men was found to have committed a burglary and was sent to jail for six months. It was Mercy, the leader of the rebellious group who later resigned and moved to another village in the Chikwawa District just north of Nsanje District. We never heard from her again, but have often prayed that the positive influences that she experienced as a member of the class of HSAs prevail for the rest of her life as one of God's special children.

Graduation plans were in the hands of the Health Inspectors, the Horticulturist and the natural leaders among the Health Surveillance Assistants. Malawians love every type of celebration, and the graduation program was a very big event and received a lot of attention and planning. This Child Survival Project was well-networked with various local, regional and national government agencies, so it was most appropriate to invite the participation of government as well as church officials in the acknowledgement of the significant accomplishment of twenty-two talented village health workers.

The students wrote an original drama of sickness and health interventions, they also practiced a song of God's hands being involved in their learning how to serve their people in a health ministry. The program supervisors organized the details of a communal meal for officials, project personnel and various representatives of the several churches that participated in the training. The invitation list brought interested people together from across the southern half of the nation. On the day of the ceremony, everyone in the program was busy cleaning and decorating the training center. As guests arrived they were seated by well dressed students and offered a basin of water and towel to wash their hands. The meal consisted of traditional *nsima*, hot chicken and vegetable relish, cabbage salad, Asian style tea with much sugar and milk, and sweet biscuits – all graciously served by the women in the class.

The local pastor offered a prayer of blessing for the meal and for the future efforts of these graduates. Ken was busy photographing the event. When the dishes were cleared away the class presented a dynamic drama that was sometimes tender and insightful into family life and alcoholism in the bush villages, and sometimes induced raucous laughter as they interwove the humor of village life. Then there were the speeches: The Horticulturist for rural agriculture in Nsanje District was a beautiful woman with a Master's degree. Her speech challenged the graduates to continue to pursue education even while they serve as Health Surveillance Assistants. She was personally a role model for such pursuit, having emerged from a very poor village in the District. There were other speeches of varying lengths: the Dutch physician from the Trinity Hospital

Catholic Parish, who had served so capably on our Advisory Committee; the Malawian Public Health Nurse who had been one of our lead instructors; and the Member of Parliament for that Region, Mr. Phinda, whose first duty it always was to praise the President-for-Life, the Kamuzu Banda. After due praise for the the Kamuzu, Mr. Phinda made the formal graduation address and presented the Ministry of Health-approved Certificates of Completion to the students. To close the event, the students sang their own song about God's Hands in rich vocal harmony.

CHAPTER 8

LET THERE BE LIGHT

The First Assignment

In order to have week-to-week contact with over 3,000 families in southern Malawi's bush country, our HSAs would need to select and train at least 25 volunteers to serve as "Mother Visitors" in their own neighborhoods. This was to be their first activity after graduation. Together, the HSAs, their instructors and I, selected the most important health and life-style messages that we must teach our Mother Visitors. The Ministry of Health provided posters and booklets ready for our use. Up until this Child Survival Project, there was simply nobody prepared to go to these highest risk villages. The messages, artists' drawings and illustrations, were in the simplest Chichewa language and had been taken from the UNICEF publication, Facts for Life, A Communication Challenge. We began with preventive messages and management of the prime killers of infants and young children: Home hygiene and Sanitation, Diarrhea Prevention and Management, and Immunizations.

Ultimately, the Mother Visitors would learn to teach and guide on:

- Malaria
- Nutrition for the Growing Child
- AIDS
- Birth Timing and Control
- Safe Motherhood
- Coughs and Colds
- Child Growth and Development
- Breastfeeding

The initial training of Mother Visitors would last two weeks, with subsequent quarterly one-week training sessions. Some villages spanned a circumference of ten miles, so it was necessary for the project to support the volunteering Mother Visitors with a place to stay and their food during the weeks of training. Since this was our HSA's first venture into training other adults, we knew that the experience would call upon their very best skills. We hoped that we had adequately taught them to be trainers. To ensure the best outcomes possible, we teamed our HSAs together to do the initial training. Together, they would plan the training experience they would deliver. Then they, as a team, would present the training to the selected volunteers in the village where one partner HSA resided. The next two weeks they would present the training to the volunteers in the other HSA's village. With this schedule for eleven teams of two in locations as distant from each other as much as 150 kilometers, Ken was kept very busy transporting team members and moving their supplies among and between villages.

Before their graduation day, the HSAa were given opportunity to make their training plans and to role model their introductory session before the entire class of HSAs. Also, before they were actually deployed to start this training, we gave them two-day training in AIDS Prevention

Education. Their teacher for this experience was named Michael Uzi. He was not only a Certified Medical Assistant, but also a very accomplished dramatist. Again, there is a cultural norm in Malawi that one of the best learning modalities is lively drama. Michael's drama was designed with the objective of changing the social customs related to sexual activities, knowing that the behaviors of acknowledged leaders would have to change first. Village people model after their Chiefs, appointed village Head Men, elected political party counselors at the village, traditional healers and midwives, pastors and priests. Traditionally, there are very few female role models.

After learning with Michael Uzi for two days, the HSAs were eager to enact one of his scripts. To depict something of the giftedness of these 22 learners, Michael spent just one-half hour with them in reviewing the story line, selecting which roles fit which HSA, and setting the outdoor stage under the tree! Four HSAs and Michael played the parts of two village women who loved and were the wives of the same man, a Village Chief; a modern foreign medical doctor, and the traditional healer.

The dramatized scenario evolved as follows: one of the women becomes ill and blames the man, who totally denied anything was wrong. The other woman lectured the man when she learned the other wife was ill, and she literally drug her husband to the medical doctor in a distant village. Disbelief and denial of HIV infection persisted even after tests revealed that the man was indeed HIV positive.

Then the traditional healer returned to their village after a long absence. He listened to the recitation by one of the wives of how so many dear friends and relatives had died of *Edze* since he had been away. The healer called both wives together with the infected Chief and told them what he had learned from trusted medical doctors in another village. He told him that from this moment on they must not have sex with anyone else and he took all three back to the modern medical doctor. Of course, the doctor confirmed to the three individuals that what their traditional healer told them is true. He tested both women and found that one was HIV positive and the other still negative. Together, the family members talked about treatment and about death and dying with the doctor and their traditional healer. In the chance and the hope that the second wife might not convert to HIV positive she agreed to not have sex with her infected husband. She knew that she needed desperately to live in order to care for the trio's several children.

The drama then depicted how the Village Chief and the healer were both committed to informing and modeling the healthiest lifestyle possible before the rest of the village. They would hope to show that just one woman for each man is the way God intended for people to live, and that this is the only way the occurrence of AIDS could be diminished among the people. The drama closed with the drama team presenting a rousing song about the horror of *Edze* and the one sure way to block its transmission. Michael's drama so inspired the Child Survival staff, that at least half of the HSAs determined that they would develop drama teams among their volunteers to carry the message everywhere in the lower Shire River valley.

The cultural norm for marriage in Malawi, at that time, was that a man should have as many wives as he could afford to keep. It goes without saying, wives usually brought their youth, two more hands, and another strong back to do the gardening, carry the water, cook the food and have many children. When a visiting man comes to the village, it was customary for the host man to present his wives so that the visitor could choose which one would give him warmth during the visit! Prostitution is part of the old Malawi way of life and as men travel from place to place to obtain work, if there was an overnight en route, they could always find warmth, food and comfort with one of the women along the way.

These cultural norms fostered AIDS as a heterosexual problem in Malawi, and at that time, studies of birth mothers at Queen Elizabeth Hospital in Blantyre showed that 24% of women in childbearing years were HIV positive. Five years later the percentage was up to 33% but seemed to be leveling off. Many entire villages have been left with only the aging grandparents and the non-infected children to care for one another. The young people, and often the brightest, have died of AIDS.

Traditionally, the funeral customs in any village demand about a week's time for all the people to mourn, bury the dead and to feast and drink *chabuka* together. It then takes about another week for the adults to sober up and get back to the work of hunting, fishing, gardening, and the cycle of life as they know it. We observed many villages coming to this mournful standstill for weeks with multiple funerals occurring nearly every day.

Training Village Mother Visitors

As HSAs began to establish their presence as responsible, mid-level village health workers, they held planning meetings with the Chiefs and Head Men. Village Health Committees were appointed by the Head Men from among acknowledged "helpers" in the neighborhoods. About half of the HSAs were women and they all sought to have some women on the Health Committees. The first task of these committees was to identify potential volunteer mother visitors who were interviewed by the HSA and ultimately, officially appointed by the Health Committee as Mother Visitors.

We had set certain criteria for the appointment of Mother Visitors. We preferred that they be women who could read and write their own language. They must not be leaving young children alone and unattended while they were in training or in the future when they would visit other families or be attending village clinics with some of their highest risk families. We soon learned, however, that this population in the bush of southernmost Malawi had very few men who were literate and sometimes no adult women who could read or write Chichewa. In such cases, the men suggested that we train the traditional midwives, and when necessary, the men who could be Mother Visitors would help with the small amount of paper work and reporting. Although the nation's President had decreed in the late 1960's that "Full Primary Schools" would exist in all areas, schools were not begun in this district until 1986. Even when primary education became available, the cultural standard was that girls do not need to read or write. After all, they need to be kept tilling the fields, transporting water on their heads, doing the laundry on a rock in the river (when the river was not dry), and having many babies. Only since 1986 had any girls been sent to school; however, the donor nations who were assisting in this "third world's" development, notified the Malawi Ministry of Education that, beginning in 1992, each classroom must be attended by girls equal to the number of boys. If equality of education for both sexes was not actively achieved, educational donor money would be cut off.

When the village people began to hear about volunteering for Child Survival work, most of them wanted to be chosen. It was good that we had some criteria for selection and that the village leaders, themselves, did the final appointing. They all seemed to be hungry to learn and thirsting for a better life.

I could not help but be especially interested in the outcomes of our two most remote villages, Misamvu and Kanyimbi. Mr. Honex Faind Phiri, HSA, chose to be stationed in Misamvu and Mr. Castings Mchiza, HSA, chose Kanyimbi because his younger brother was a primary school teacher there. Both of these men were married and had wives and children about 100 kilometers distant in the valley. Both young men had experienced some successes in farming and business, hence it was an unusual sacrifice for them to make to choose these distant locales.

Theirs was the first scheduled training for volunteer Mother Visitors, and I had made a commitment to attend the completion ceremonies for as many of these groups as possible. It was a particularly hot day as I drove with Supervising HI, James, and the 140 kilometers from Ngabu to Misanvu. The classes had been conducted in an unused classroom in the Primary School. The final oral examination for the Mother Visitors was to be administered by James, followed by speeches of congratulation by village leaders and the HSA team teachers, and a festive communal dinner of goat meat stew with vegetables and *nsima*.

As 25 pairs of dusty, bare, black feet entered the room I was impressed by the wonderful courtesy they each observed. Bowing graciously to their leaders and me at the doorway, they took their seats at good classroom desks. By presidential edict, no class or formal meeting ever begins without a prayer to the Creator-God. HSA, Honex designated one of the men to pray (there were only 2 women in the class of Volunteer Mother Visitors – both of them traditional midwives). The designated man asked the people to stand and bow their heads, and it was about this time, with the deep resonant voice of this man thanking God for the Child Survival opportunity, that I began to fill up with tears. This is the beginning of results, here in this faraway place, with these wonderful people, excited and happy to serve their own.

I could understand some of the Chichewa words in James' oral examination. As each student was addressed, he or she stood up, erect, and addressed their answer, "Sir, ..." As each one confidently responded to question after question, they demonstrated how well prepared in understanding of the purposes of the project, their anticipated roles and the health messages, interventions and actions they could give. As I listened and watched, the hot sun was beating down on that tin roof and brick walls, and flies began to buzz around our faces. Brushing them off, I jotted down some of my impressions and those moving thoughts became a poem, entitled *Jesus Christ in Misamvu.* Although I have used this poem many times since that day, I have never been impressed to edit it. Here is how it goes:

Jesus walked the dusty trails to Misamvu today;
Bare, black feet on the thorny ground, under the African sun.
He came in the heart of His child, Mr. Phiri --
He, Who risked all to save all people, came
Into Mr. Phiri's heart, to call him, also, to a certain risk;
The risk of leaving his home and family, in order to serve;
And the risk of rejection by those whom he came to serve.

Jesus talked to the people in Misamvu today;
And the people said, "you are welcome!
Did you bring us medicine?"
But Jesus, in Mr. Phiri, said, "I give you better than medicine;
I give you myself, to live among you and to teach you,
That your children might not die."
"I come to show you a new and better way;
I want to make Disciples* of you.
Then you, too, can show and teach a better way."

Jesus taught His disciples in Misamvu today;
Those who responded to His call; and
The love of God was carried to this furthest outpost of Malawi;
To forever, change the hearts and lives of His children there.

Now, a child cries out in fever and pain, and
A mother's anguished look appears.
Jesus responds through His disciples who are
listening, treating, encouraging, teaching, and touching.
The mother responds to Him by listening, learning,
cleansing and patiently rehydrating her child.
And the child then responds to Him with laughter...
playing in the sunshine.

And the village people begin to clean the entire village,
Protecting their water supply; planting better gardens,
Teaching and learning from one another, and
Praising *Mulungu,* the One God who made them,
and called them
to a more abundant life!

Jesus prayed in Misamvu today; the prayer gratefully yielding
these children to the Father's care.
Jesus lives in the hearts of many in Misamvu today,
because He came in the heart of one man.
*Child Survival Volunteers

Mr. Mchiza's family had no plans to join him in mountainous Kanyimbi. The older children were in school and *mayi* (mother) Mchiza was an excellent manager in overseeing the planting, growing and harvesting of their cotton, maize and guar bean crops.

Mr. Phiri's wife was much younger and they had a young child eleven months old. They seemed very happy as they first moved all the family *katundu* up and out to Misamvu. After only about a month, mother, and young son joined Mr. Phiri and Ken in the old blue Toyota when all was ready for them in the Misamvu house. As Ken drove up through the ebony forest, he became increasingly concerned at the severe coughing, strangling, and crying of the baby. He suggested that they turn around and go back to the Kalema Parish Hospital for some medical help, but the parents declined, saying they were sure the baby would be all right just as soon as the motion of the car was past. Ken again asked as they were putting things away into that little brick home, if they would please allow him to take mother and baby back to the hospital about 70 kilometers away. Again, they refused, and about dusk, Ken left to maneuver the Land Cruiser down the rugged footpath, just barely wide enough for the 4-wheel drive Toyota. He felt sadness as he brought the vehicle back to the tarmac and past the Parish Hospital. One week later, as the jungle drums brought the message, we learned that the suffering baby died the next morning and even the traditional healer in Misamvu village recognized the condition as whooping cough.

Although this child was still breast feeding and thus receiving disease-fighting antibodies from his mother, he had not completed the important infant immunization for diphtheria, pertussis, and tetanus (DPT). Needless to say, the mother and father were devastated. The young mother said she could not stay in that remote village any longer and she returned to her parents' home. She hinted at leaving her husband forever and finding a man who could give her strong babies that would not die at the least infection. Ultimately she did divorce Mr. Phiri, but he determined that he had made this commitment to his God and his people and he would stay on alone, if need be.

The Creativity of Dorika

Before we left our Washington, D.C. orientation course, we received an anonymous gift of just over $100.00 to be used however, we thought would be useful in our work. The money just stayed in our bank while we listened and learned from these new friends. Rhoda and Jessie were always busy helping others although they had very few kwacha of their own. Both were leaders in the women's organization, known as "Dorika," at their home church in Ngabu. It was easy to see that the word, Dorika, came from the New Testament scriptural model of community service and a woman called Dorcas. As we observed them ministering to the elderly, the orphans, the burnout victims and the very sick in this small community, we wondered how to help them. Occasionally, I met with them in their monthly meetings under the trees. How I enjoyed sitting on their grass mats, learning their songs, hearing their testimonies and praying with these beautiful women! It finally occurred to us that they needed some kind of income generating activity (IGA) in order to better serve their community. And the seed money was resting in our bank!

The Dorika women were so excited when we asked how they might like to earn money, if they had a little money to start with! We did not tell them how much! They took turns suggesting everything from growing gardens (what about the drought years?... they asked themselves), raising and herding cattle, crocheting caps for women to wear to church, and finally coming to consensus that they would have a ready market for school-age children's clothing. You see, children in southern Malawi are seldom seen in clothing until they reach school age, where at least the boys wear shirts and short pants and the girls wear blouses and skirts. Don't ask about underwear! Remember it is very warm here! Most families take pride in sending their children off to school, but many have no money to buy clothes. However, they will happily trade a chicken or a pig for clothing found for sale under the trees in the village market.

Yes! The women would have their very own Income Generating Activity (IGA) to create children's clothing, sewn by hand, and sold/traded in the market for *kwacha* or food. Then they would have no difficulty in selling the chicken or pig, or even produce received in the bargaining. Then, we asked them to brainstorm their goals for using the funds. They quickly came to agreement, for they knew the needs of their community well. Then, we told them there was enough *kwacha* available from our friends in America to buy the various types of fabric, the scissors, needles, and thread. They could begin right away! Many of these women did not own a pair of scissors, let alone ever held a needle in their hands, but they were willing to learn. One of the Dorika leaders was married to a village tailor and she knew that with his help, she could teach the rest, as the supplies became available.

The Dorika leaders involved their church Treasurer and the church Board members so that there was accountability for money received and money spent. We cut the check for a bit more than we had received in Washington, D.C. and they held a lovely presentation ceremony at the church. Their written goals included:

- To help elderly people obtain medicine when they cannot afford it;
- To assist families whose thatch huts burn (as happens frequently) to re-establish their homes;
- To pay for school fees for AIDS orphans who are living with their relatives.

Everyone in the church - over 400 adult members - felt ownership in their own Dorika's IGA! Six months later, they had sold everything they had created, and had three times the amount of money they began with - in the bank! They invited me to attend their monthly meetings, sitting on bamboo mats on the ground; singing their songs; sharing their family stories; their joys, the hardships, and their faith in Mulungu! People with nearly nothing, celebrating everything!

Cross-cultural Partners – The Asian Family Merchants

With our location just about 15 degrees above the equator, sunset and sunrise always came "early" and suddenly! It was suddenly dark between six and seven o'clock in the evening; and it was suddenly very light (and hot!) about twelve hours later. Often, when the sun went down, so did the electrical supply on Saopa Road in Ngabu. We both enjoy reading and letter writing time in the evenings, so decided the next time we were shopping in Blantyre we would try to purchase a Coleman-type gasoline lantern. Usually, one of us made the trip to the commercial city once a week to purchase supplies for the HSAs and the office and to replenish our groceries from one of the nation's two, government-owned, super markets.

Busy Haile Selassie Boulevard in Blantyre housed shops specializing in everything from new Mercedes-Benz automobiles to freshly butchered beef. Traffic was a noisy, horn-blowing, shouting, bumper-to-bumper experience, and parking was nearly impossible. So, for a Coleman lantern, I left the Toyota Land Cruiser at the ADRA headquarters and enjoyed the walk downtown. The closer I came to Haile Selassie Blvd. the more closely packed were the pedestrians. Some carried huge banana stalks on their heads to take them to a place on the shady side of the street and hawk them for a few tambalas each. Others were impeccably dressed business people rushing to or from their modern office buildings. Still others were street people who had no home, but wandered the streets, begging and perhaps finding a relative's mud hut on the edge of the city for nighttime safety. My sense of cultural shock never really dimmed, it always was a sensory roller coaster. From joy in the happy faces of many, to sorrow and pity for the crippled and destitute beggars. Many of them polio victims with the added baggage of AIDS and/or alcoholism. The begging grandmothers with "river-blindness" from water born parasites, challenged my senses on this tearful walk downtown.

I had spotted several "hardware" stores earlier and headed directly to the first one I remembered. I noticed with excitement that right there in the window was a real Coleman lantern! As I entered, I found a friendly East-Indian shopkeeper dressed in the long white robe and white crochet skullcap of the Muslim Mosque assistant. As the owner of the store, he greeted me graciously, but said that he was about to leave for his Friday noon prayer responsibilities at the Mosque. However, he said he would take a moment to help me. When I asked about the lantern, he quickly indicated that I must walk with him a few doors further down the street to his son's hardware store where I could purchase a lantern and everything else I would need for "the best price in Malawi." Father Ashid led me into a tiny shop about 10 feet wide and 30 feet long, with high ceilings lined with shelving and hooks laden with merchandise all the way to the very high ceiling. Black Malawians were busily assisting other customers, and a healthy cacophony of Chichewa language bargaining almost drowned the racket from the street. A handsome, smiling, young man about 25 bowed deeply to his father and to me and I met Hamed for the first time.

Both men wanted to know who I was, where I came from and if I was affiliated in any way with Malamulo Hospital in Makwasa, rural Thyolo District, about 70 kilometers distant. When I explained my mission work with ADRA, they seemed very pleased; but were a bit disappointed that as a health care worker, my relationship with the Adventist flagship hospital in the Malawi bush country was only indirect. They both praised the hospital, stating they preferred it very much over the Blantyre Adventist Hospital (or any other government or private hospital in that city) for its high quality of health and illness care rendered by the multi-national team of health professionals there. Mr. Ashid indicated that there was no other hospital in the nation that his large extended family would even consider using, even with the distant drive to get there. He and his family made routine visits to the physicians there, had necessary surgery there, and even delivered some of their babies at Malamulo. He also shared with me that he and his father before him had made significant contributions to improve, equip, and maintain the 100-year old health care center.

Suddenly Father Ashid excused himself as he directed his son to be very good to me and give me the "best prices in Malawi" for whatever my needs might be. Father left quickly for Friday's work at the Mosque as the call to Moslem prayer sounded above the routine noises of the city.

I purchased the Coleman lantern for half the price listed on the one I had seen in Father's shop. Then, I decided to check out pricing on bicycle parts because I had purchased a variety of parts elsewhere just that very day and I could compare. So my purchases included a bike tire, spokes for the wheels, and several other items. Indeed, to my delight I found they must indeed be the best prices in Malawi! Everything was from 25% to 75% less than my earlier, similar purchases elsewhere.

We made many trips to Blantyre with nearly every trip including the last stop at Hamed's Hardware. Our HSAs and the three professional leaders were overjoyed as the 24 project bicycles arrived from the manufacturer in India and the 3 Suzuki motorcycles came in from the Republic of South Africa. The Suzuki "Ag Bikes" were issued to the Health Inspectors and the Horticulturist but remained the property of ADRA. However, the Advisory Committee recommended that as an incentive toward good bicycle maintenance, every Health Surveillance Assistant who stayed with the project would ultimately own their own bike. Another role for my husband, Ken, emerged: teaching safe cycling and bike maintenance to everyone! Many of our project staff had never held a screwdriver in their hand, let alone ridden a bicycle! The three professional team leaders also had much to learn from Ken and the operational manuals about the care and handling of their motorized Ag Bikes.

On one trip I, showed Hamed a longer list of needed hardware and then asked him if he also carried watering cans for gardens. I had priced these handcrafted tin cans with spray spouts and needed 120 of them for our demonstration kitchen gardens. Again, Hamed's wares were half the cost of the same items elsewhere. That day we talked a long time about the Child Survival Project. He seemed fascinated with the training we had done with young Malawians, and the ways in which they were teaching and leading hundreds of families into a healthier lifestyle.

I was fascinated with his stories of how he is a third generation Malawian who had graduated from university in England where he also held citizenship. He told me how he had learned to love the hardware business from working with his father, and of his contacts all over the world to obtain anything his customers could need. His face fell as he described the tragic automobile accidental death of his younger brother, Mizha, and how his mother had been severely depressed for the past two years since Mizha's death. I asked if I might meet his mother sometime, and he just beamed and said he would make sure of it.

As his "*bambos*" loaded the good old blue Toyota Land Cruiser, Hamed said to me, "I honor you for what you are doing for my people and my country. I will always see that whatever you need from me is the very best and at my cost in price. Oh, how I wish I could do what you do for my people! The only thing I know how to do is to make money!" Suddenly, I knew there was something very special about this young man, and I believe it was the Holy Spirit who impressed me to respond: "Hamed, thank you for your appreciation of my mission. While I was born to teach and to heal, you were called to be the fine businessman that you are. I do not know how to make money; I do know how to teach health. You are not a teacher; but you are a businessman. But I think we hold some of the same values in common. We both desire a better life for the people in Malawi's villages. You know that the limited money that I spend to keep our project functioning is not my money. It is God's money. You are Muslim; I am Christian, but I think we serve the same God, the Creator of the universe. And whenever you help me stretch God's money further to provide for this service project, we are partnering with God!" Hamed's eyes widened and his smile also, as he said, "I guess I have never thought of it in that way!" He shook my hand warmly, bowed and we said goodbye.

During one of my visits to Hamed's Hardware, I was delighted to meet Hamed's beautiful mother, Ramina. She was dressed in an elegant East Indian dress, with a scarf that covered her head, and was most gracious to me offering me tea, which we enjoyed together in the back of that crowded, noisy store. I complimented her on her handsome and brilliant son, noting that I had observed his love and respect toward her, and related a bit of my experience in getting acquainted with her husband and her son. She told me of the sadness that had enveloped her life since her other son's death. She had her own women and children's fine clothing shop right on Haile Selassie Blvd., but because of her grief, she just could not open it any more. Last year's new clothing was still on the racks, the windows shuttered and the door locked.

But her eyes sparkled as she told me of her plan to visit England where so many of her family members live. The purpose of her visit would be to choose a bride for her son, Hamed. In my Western way, I asked when she and Hamed would be leaving, and she responded, "Oh, but you must understand. In my culture, it is the mother of the young man who chooses his bride. He has nothing to do with it." She explained that she had been corresponding with some of her Asian friends, and the mother of the young woman had already approved of the union of the two families. All that Ramina would be doing on her visit to London would be to visit the young woman and her mother, arrange for a very large engagement party for women only, celebrate the de facto engagement, and return with many elaborate gifts for her family. Her son would not even see a photo or video of his bride-to-be until she returned from England. The wedding would be performed in England a few months later, and another ceremony would take place when the couple eventually returns to home in Blantyre.

I could see that powerful healing for Ramina's deep depression was available and already at work in her planning for her son's future. When she was picked up by her driver in a Mercedes-Benz sedan, she waved happily and promised to serve Ken and me a truly East Indian feast soon.

Hamed seemed very pleased at my meeting with his mother, and then shared a secret with me. Before he did so, he made me promise to never tell his mother! That was difficult for me to do, but I promised! He had just returned from one week in Capetown, South Africa, where he had one last fling as a single man. He and a good male friend had pre-arranged dates in Capetown with two American co-eds attending the University there. He took me to the back office to show me the color photos of their dates at the beach, at the restaurants and nightclubs, at the yacht races as well as some beauty spots of that city.

Then we began loading from ten to twenty hand-made tin watering cans in the Land Cruiser, filling available space up to the ceiling of the vehicle; the cans rattling and banging all the way down the rugged 70-kilometer distance to the sunroom (*khonde*) in our home on Saopa Road. This transport of cans took place every week until all 120 were stacked in our *khonde* to be picked up and strapped onto Horticulturist, Davis Mchawa's Suzuki motorcycle. At first, I wondered how these cans would ever reach their destinations, but this dedicated teacher made sure I was at home when he loaded the second batch! He showed me how he used strips of rubber from old tire inner tubes to lash these important tools to the motorcycle. That Suzuki rattled and banged all the way down into the bush villages, (sometimes 100 kilometers distant) where one by one, the cans reached their destinations! Davis was living proof of our saying, "Where there is a will, there is a way!" He was also known as "the Can-do man"!

Our relationships with this Asian merchant family

blossomed as they came to know Ken and met some of our project leaders. Eventually Ramina made her visit to England staying about two months. When she returned she and Ashid invited us to their modern home for a marvelous Chambo fish dinner (a type of bass harvested commercially from the abundance of Lake Malawi) with all of the East Indian accompaniments. After dinner, with Hamed present, Ramina showed us the color video of Hamed's betrothed, Druszhabin, and the lavish engagement party that her family and Ramina had given in London. The bride-to-be was just sixteen, but well educated and very beautiful. Her party dress was colorful, elegantly styled organza and she was attended by dozens of equally beautiful young women who presented her with lavish gifts, some from the Orient, and others from the United Kingdom or the United States. This was the equivalent of the most lavish bridal shower one could imagine and all these gifts were added to the traditional bridal dowry.

As we viewed the 90-minute video, Hamed was visibly excited and pleased with Druszhabin, his mother's choice for his wife. He would nudge Ken and ask, "Isn't she just marvelous?" Of course, both of us affirmed his perceptions, but then Hamed would proclaim another superlative of her beauty, her family background, and his undying love for her. But they had never met personally! The wedding was planned for a London Mosque, almost a year in the future. Of course, Mother Ramina and Father Ashid were very satisfied with Hamed's responses and the plans for this union of two fine Muslim families of East Indian descent. The next day, Ramina opened her clothing shop for the first time in almost two years. She did it for me, but also she knew it would be a further healing step to regain her energy and emerge out of the darkness of depression and grief. Of course, I found just what I needed – a gift of clothing for a newborn baby in our Saopa Road neighborhood. We felt a warm friendship with the entire Asian family and as our time in Malawi grew shorter, we promised to maintain contact through their modern communication resources: FAX, phone, postal services, and e-mail. The technology for communication was there but not always functioning. Communications were often shut down because of failures of the electrical system that obtained power from the huge waterfalls on the Shire River

CHAPTER 9

LIGHTS IN THE DARKNESS

From Vision to Reality

With 22 HSAs deployed and serving over 12,000 families with children under three or a pregnant mother, we felt real joy and a certain sense of accomplishment within just 22 months of our arrival. Each deployed HSA had established Village Health Committees in all the assigned villages and recruited and trained approximately 25 Village Mother Visitors. Regular "wellness" clinics were set up in most remote areas to assess babies and identify those with malnutrition so we could provide enriched porridge formula or they could be referred to the special nutrition clinics operated by the two Catholic parishes. In collaboration with the District Health Officer, the Health Inspectors picked up and delivered immunization supplies to HSAs for use in the weekly clinics. All the project staff understood the principle of the "cold chain" process for protecting the vaccines with dry ice, wet ice, and/or refrigeration. In most instances, dry ice kept the immunization pack cold until the HI delivered it to the destination clinic (usually held under a tree). Some villages used the kerosene refrigerators at the local bar, by special arrangements with the bar owner!

Village Mother Visitors (VMVs) participated in monthly training events conducted by their HSA and/or the Health Inspector assigned to their area. These VMVs conducted regularly scheduled home visits, teaching sanitation, personal hygiene, child spacing, AIDS protection, prevention, and management of diarrhea, and other health messages. With these consistent visits, teaching and demonstrations, families gained confidence and were gradually willing to participate in the group clinics where the HSAs taught other preventive health subjects and gave mothers a chance to ask questions. Ken and I personally visited nearly every locale to observe and participate in assisting village leaders to take an active part in working to maintain and improve their supply of clean water, and in supporting the work of the village health committee, and registering births, since there was no national system for Vital Statistics at that time!

Is Any Moonsmoke Clearing Away Yet?

Both Ken and I had suffered through the ravages of the malarial parasites even though we had been faithful in taking our preventive medicine and using every imaginable mosquito protection. The entire lower Shire River valley where we lived and worked had many fertile swamps that could not be drained except by extreme government measures. The edges of these swampy areas were great producers of foodstuffs for the entire nation (and some for export) in the good years The *anopheles mosquito* thrives in these swamps and achieve their daily blood feast from animals and humans, leaving behind a deposit of the potent parasites that cause high mortality for children and elderly. Malaria parasites rather quickly become resistant to new medicines, and ultimately, Ken and I succumbed. We lost considerable weight and energy with this insult. Also, the sheer enormity of our responsibilities was taking its toll on our energies, both physically and mentally. When those responsibilities were not consistently supported by accurate accounting and allocation of the project resources, my body responded with a pyloric gastric ulcer, identified by X-rays ordered by our good friend Dr. Peter Jaggi at Blantyre Adventist Hospital. When Malaria struck us, it was Dr. Peter and his wonderful wife, Vrenni, who insisted they set up a hospital room in their home for Ken and me to receive essential intravenous therapy and nursing care. The hospital was just across the road from their home, so nurses came and went from their duty stations to care for us. At the time of this writing, we understand that Peter and Vrenni serve as Country Directors for ADRA International in Kabul, Afghanistan.

We had served in Malawi for almost 18 months when the planned evaluation of the Child Survival Project was completed and the report received. Two American physicians knowledgeable in tropical medicine and international health policy joined the Malawi evaluation team of both government and non-governmental health professionals to perform on-site evaluation of the work of the project staff, to learn responses from village leaders, and to measure outcomes of the first and second years of the project. It was a great satisfaction to me as I received the evaluation report that indicated that we were achieving most of our goals in a very time- and labor-efficient way. Of course, evaluation pointed out areas of the project that needed special attention in order to be more successful. Evaluation team members had seen with their own eyes the difference that health education makes in the project villages since they had begun to receive the day-to-day services of their own Health Committee, the HSAs, and their own Village Mother Visitors. THEN, it was time to go home!

The Malawi ADRA Director sought and found a fine Medical Assistant working in an ambulatory clinic, to which I would provide project management orientation and a sense of the thrills and chills of this very dynamic operation. The potential new manager was very pleased with the house on Saopa Road for it was bigger and much better he and his wife had ever enjoyed. His wife was a Registered Nurse but was experiencing a very severe Diabetic crisis, a condition that was very difficult to manage. She reluctantly approved of the major change in their residence, her husband's work, and the distance they would be from her trusted medical advisors in the city. Although the new Project Manager shared much of my enthusiasm for the project, I could see that the scenario might not work out for them. And it did not. In only a few weeks after we were gone, another American woman came to Ngabu to manage the project.

One afternoon during our last few weeks in Ngabu, I was working at the computer in the project office when there was a knock on the glass door and four men I had never seen before entered. They introduced themselves as the elders of a small Adventist church in Mphonde Village not far away. They said that one of our project HSAs, Mr. Castings Mchiza, was also their church treasurer and that he had suggested that they come to me for assistance. I asked them to be seated and moved my chair from behind the desk, so that we sat together in a semi-circle. Only one of the men spoke any English, but he carefully laid out their reason for being there. The problem was that although they are an organized body of believers in Jesus Christ, they had no church building. They told me that their village is one of the poorest in terms of individual and group income. They asserted that they desperately want a church building in which to worship and told how they had already made enough bricks to build a big church and enough more bricks to sell. The only reason they were there was to plead that ADRA, or *bambo* Ken and *mayi* Bee, themselves, would help them build their church.

Here I was again, appealing in my mind to my Heavenly Father to guide me in my responses to these precious, people. As for ADRA building churches, I knew that was out of the question since ADRA is a "capacity builder" in developing communities, but does not directly support denominational church construction. I had no idea where resources would come from otherwise. So, I complimented them on sharing with me their deep desire to serve the Lord better through a building where others could be joining them as they see the building emerge. There was no church of any denomination for miles around Mphonde Village. When I asked them if they had requested assistance from the national Seventh-day Adventist organization, the Malawi Union Mission, they replied that they had not. I then encouraged them to do so, and explained to them that sometimes, the larger organization might negotiate the provision of "matching" funds for such worthy projects. They shared that they had even gone so far as to pour the concrete footings for their church and the building they would construct would seat over 500 people! These were spokespersons and leaders for a body of about 75 members presently! They invited us to come and see the location they had laid out. My promise to them was that we must pray together that day for God's will to be done and then my husband and I would lift their need to God as we go home and just see what God would do when many voices are raised to Him on behalf of this noble plan. Although I felt quite helpless in my responses, nevertheless I felt a thrill that somehow God had big plans for Mphonde Village. After praying with these gentlemen, we shook hands and they left. In a few days, Ken visited Mphonde and found that, indeed, they had laid out a very professional building scheme with footings in place and huge piles of newly-burnt bricks waiting. His only reassurance to the representatives of the church community was that we would pray to our Heavenly Father for the help that they needed.

There were many sweet relationships that would be affected by our leaving, so we were not too surprised when the community brought a "farewell party" to our home one evening. Over thirty members of the community came bearing simple gifts of carved ebony or malumba wood, fabrics and other small objects of esteem. It was in the midst of this party that the Dorika leader came to me and knelt beside me as the room went silent so she could give her final report on the sewing and income generating activity. She recounted the number of children's garments that had been made and sold. She told of the families that had been helped, especially the school fees that were paid on behalf of AIDS orphans and their grandparent-caregivers. When she finished, everyone in the room clapped and shouted for the good work of the Ngabu Dorika. Then, in a strong, sweet voice, this woman leader spoke to Ken and me, "These clothing items that we sold were all made, as you know, without the help of a sewing machine. Our fingers move slowly, and we could sell many more items if we had a treadle sewing machine! When you go home to the U.S.A., we know that you will send us a sewing machine, so we can do so much better and earn even more money to help the needy people in Ngabu." We promised to pray about how to provide them with a treadle sewing machine, and then led the whole group in prayer for their continued blessing and for a safe trip home for we two *izungus.*

Little did we realize that they would hold us accountable for that prayer! Six months after we were back home in Idaho, we received a letter from the Ngabu Dorika asking that we provide them with that special sewing machine. So, we telephoned to Hamed, our favorite merchant, to see if he could obtain a good, used treadle machine and he answered affirmatively He even delivered the machine, without charge, the 70 kilometers distant, to these dedicated Dorika women!.

During our last few days in the house on Saopa Road, Ken was very busy constructing a shipping crate from hand-hewn lumber from the hardwood tree called *Malumba.* The crate needed to contain the several items of furniture made from the Shire River reeds and grasses that we had purchased for our living room there. When it was finished, the crate looked like a double-decker casket! Ken loves fine woodworking, his discovery of Malumba and Ebony was something that he could cherish. Since it is against Malawi and some international law to export this wood, but legal to use it for utilitarian purposes, we could make our own shipping crate and then use it for artistic purposes in Ken's shop at home in the U.S. It was indeed, utilitarian – very heavy and very sturdy. When the day arrived to load the crate and all the rest of our *katundu,* Ken and our faithful watchman, McDonald Ntupa were struggling to inch it from the sun room, onto planks and into the utility trailer when that "Angel Man" Akim Kafukiza showed up. His lift was all they needed to ease that huge crate into the trailer and then Akim and his wife, Farmessa, climbed into the back seat of the Land Cruiser so they could accompany us to Blantyre. Somehow, the people of Ngabu knew the hour we would be leaving, and they lined the roads and the tarmac highway to shout and wave goodbye to us. No, our eyes were not dry for several minutes as Ken kept the rig pointed north on the road. The first stop in the city was at the shipping vender's dock that required a couple of hours of documentation and payments. Then we visited the ADRA headquarters office, the hospital and its campus, and several of the homes of hospital staff, to say goodbye. Although we had done our best to prepare for the time of leaving, it was still very heart wrenching because of the relationships of love and respect that we had enjoyed – and even struggled through – the past two years.

Some of the sweetest and saddest moments of leaving came when we arrived for dinner at the ADRA Director's home to find all of the ADRA staff there, with time for loving one another and reminiscing. We had worked with these folks for nearly two years and had come to love them as brothers and sisters. It was a pleasure to get better acquainted with the newest member of the ADRA team. At last, here was the qualified accountant ADRA needed from the start! He had set up an acceptable cost accounting system to track all the various funds that came to ADRA-Malawi where there had never been such a system. The lack of accounting had opened the door for the enormous, illegal drain of not only Adventist funds but funds received from several governments including the United States, Canada, and Denmark at that time. Our painful, whistle-blowing action finally had paid off!

We were astounded that evening when the team presented us with an elegant "memory banner" that hangs in our home The banner was hand woven especially for us by the residents of the government Home for Physically Handicapped People. On a background of hand-woven white cotton thread, is woven a pink map of Malawi with a fourth of its surface showing up as blue Lake Malawi, and the ADRA insignia woven into the southernmost tip in our Nsanje District project locale, along with our names "Bee and Ken Jarrell, Child Survival Volunteers, 1990-1992". We were moved to tears, for we even had a sense of guilt at leaving when we had only given the project a good start. As this banner hangs against the stairwell in our home, we are reminded that in Christ, our weaknesses became His enabling strength as He guided us through those beginning years and used others to complete the work as they followed in our early, halting footsteps.

ADRA usually sends its volunteers home via the reverse route of the way they travel to these far away appointments. However, Ken and I found a travel agency in the

Netherlands that is operated by Catholic Nuns especially for Christian missionaries. By careful planning we arranged air travel home that would complete a "trip around the world" for less money than the boring flight home that ADRA would arrange from Lilongwe, the capitol of Malawi, to Amsterdam, London, Washington, D.C., Denver and finally to Boise. It was quite an adventure and only the highlights follow.

Leaving Lilongwe, we stopped in Nairobi staying overnight in a downtown hotel and were accosted by a would-be thief as we went shopping for a camera that would work. Ken's good camera had given up in the bush of Nsanje District heat. Well the stealthy thief rushed me from behind and was able to slip my wristwatch off, but dropped it as he fled when I screamed! We would not have seen him drop it, but two natives nearby had seen the fiasco, and gently came to us, picking up the watch on the way and apologizing for the behavior of one of their people. As we thought about that, we wondered if that had happened someplace in the U.S., would anybody have cared? From Nairobi we took a week's guided safari journey going southeast through the Kenya plains and game preserves right to the base of majestic Mt. Kilimanjaro. What a thrill it was, moment by exciting moment, up close and very personal: giraffes, exotic birds, water buffalo, wildebeest, hartebeest, zebra, lions, elephants, monkeys and baboons, impala and half a dozen other species of antelope. Most interesting of all, was meeting some of the handsome and brightly clad Masai tribal people and learning that the Kenya government has assigned to them the management of the enormous game preserve that joins with the Kalihari Desert of Tanzania. It was obvious that they are achieving excellent results in protecting the elephants from ivory poachers, in allowing quality hotels to locate near water holes without disturbing the game habitat, and in supporting themselves through artistic achievements in silkscreen prints and superb woodcarvings.

At the end of our safari we stayed overnight in a beautiful beach hotel on the shore of the Indian Ocean about 25 miles south of the city of Mombasa. When our taxi took us to the Mombasa airport the next morning, he apologized for taking us the long way to the airport. He told us that last night there had been a street battle between Christians and Muslims in downtown Mombasa where a number of people had been killed and the city was very nervous. The flight from Mombasa to Nairobi arrived just in time to transfer from Kenya Airlines to Pakistani Airlines and fly to Karachi.

The Gulf War with Iraq had just ended and we were aware that Pakistan was not a totally friendly place for Americans to be, so we prayed for special guidance and protection for our 18-hour stopover in Karachi. Well, the government agents quickly ushered us to a private detention area as we deplaned. Our area was an 8' by 10' space with two narrow cots, two chairs, and tiny table, with a toilet down the hall, past similar spaces. We were told not to try to leave without asking the soldier at the gate to the area. To confirm our flight arrangements, the soldier went with us. Flight seats were confirmed for the next morning, but they applied a hefty surcharge on the baggage that accompanied us. What to do? We seldom carry much cash with us and they would not accept the American dollars that we had. So Ken stayed behind with our carry-on baggage in our "space" while another soldier was assigned to walk about a block away to the Pakistan bank to obtain Pakistani dollars in the proper amount to pay what we thought was a very unfair surcharge. En route, the soldier accompanying me made a couple of veiled threats that if I did not tip him properly, something bad might happen. I offered a silent prayer and pretended I did not understand what he was saying. I changed the subject to ask him about his family and by the time we reached the guard at our space, he was still telling me about beautiful children, I think. I was very glad that I could feign total ignorance about his demand for money from me. And we were greatly relieved when the noisy, sleepless night was past, morning arrived, and we were safely aboard a big jet from Thailand Airlines.

Arrival in beautiful Bangkok was uneventful where we found the Adventist Hospital and the guest quarters we had reserved. After finding some breakfast items in the cafeteria there, we crashed to sleep most of the day. The administrator of the hospital lived adjacent to our guest rooms, so when we went to thank him for the hospitality, I was amazed to learn that he had been a medical student at Loma Linda University when I was there in Nursing Education 40 years earlier. Then a woman dropped in whom I had known in my first year at college in Walla Walla, Washington. I am always impressed at how the "family of God" spreads around the world, and you are with old friends when you least expect it!

The temples and treasures of Bangkok are too beautiful and interesting to miss even during a short stay, so we stepped outside the hospital campus intending to catch a cab and ask for a quick tour of the city. Just as we did so, a beautiful Thai woman stepped between us and the cab driver, asking us if we would like a personal tour of the city with her and her friend, a handsome native standing near his Volvo at the curb. She explained that she is a Registered Nurse, had done some graduate studies at Loma Linda, and had seen us in the cafeteria early that morning. She indicated that one cannot trust the cabbies in Bangkok and that she and her friend would be pleased to host us for as long as we had the time! What a wonderful whirlwind tour we had with these two people who seemed like angels to us! We saw amazingly beautiful temples, monuments and the royal family residences throughout a city that seems to be laced with canals. When we offered American dollars as they dropped us off back at the hospital guesthouse, they totally refused. As they taught us more of the Bangkok social system and culture, we knew that we were experiencing a very rare privilege with new friends that were sent by a God who cares about us!

China Airlines took us to Taipei, Taiwan, via a refueling stop in Tokyo. Our friends at the Adventist Hospital in downtown Taipei had reserved a beautiful room for us in the nearly new Grand Hotel. We luxuriated there just long enough to sleep, take a meal or two, and risk the cab drivers there to show us Taipei by night. So, we enjoyed our first ever Mongolian Barbecue and then our cabbie-escort took us to the section of the city that non-citizens usually do not see. We visited a Buddhist temple and watched people burning incense and praying. It made us very sad to realize that millions on this planet pray to a god who is dead. The escort asked us if we had strong stomachs. We said that probably Africa had prepared us for most anything! What he led us to is still vividly burnt into my memory. On a wood rack at eye level, hung live cobra snakes by tethers just back of their flared heads. They were being milked for their venom by a man who made appropriate comments to the crowd that seemed to say in Chinese: "Step right up! Get your blood boiling for love as you drink the power of the Cobra"!. The venom was squirted into small "shot glasses" over which potent liquor was poured. This delicacy was then served at a very high price, as a powerful aphrodisiac to natives seated in the background at romantic, candle-lit tables with incense burners. We understood that ultimately the cobras would be killed, the skins marketed and the meat sold as a delicacy. It did not take very long for Ken and me to get back in that cab! It was hard to get to sleep that night in the Grand Hotel.

The next morning early, we took a tram up the steep hillsides to a teahouse, where we sampled various types of tea and left with a nice assortment to take home. And then it was time to really head for home!

We boarded China Airlines again for the flight to

Honolulu and on to a condo on Maui for a few days to shrug off culture shock. It seemed wonderful to be where everyone speaks English again. Until that day, going through customs in Hawaii, I had not realized how much psychic energy is required to understand and communicate with people of other cultures and languages. We both needed the relaxation that simply surrounded us on U.S. soil and in those enchanted islands. It was fun to bask in the sun, to play in the surf, to snorkel among so many gorgeous fish, watch the catamarans come and go, and view the sun going down beyond the palm trees. I think we flew to Los Angeles via United Airlines and were met by family and friends there. There was so much to tell, and yet we felt we could not really verbalize what Africa had meant to us, let alone what we might have meant to Africa. In God's great scheme of things in His plan for this planet, our efforts seemed just microscopic as having any real impact or influence. But, still we loved being loved by our family folks in the L.A. area.

Another quick flight took us right into beautiful downtown Boise, Idaho, and a whole host of family and friends, once again. How sweet it was! Our home had been kept in great condition by the young couple leasing it. They also took wonderful care of our dog, Sky. Sky recognized us, but seemed very confused as she tried to divide her loyalties between her new family and us, the old family. The "double-decker" hand made wooden shipping crate did not arrive for about two months as it had to be shipped via the water route. Everything arrived in good order, and we soon settled into some sort of routine that some would call "retirement."

Our hearts and minds continually felt the tug of Malawi, but we knew that we had given our best and highest while there and felt it was time for younger people to continue the good work that was begun. We left behind the 22 Health Surveillance Assistants, each of whom had trained at least

25 Volunteer Village Mother Visitors (VMVs), making a literal "army" of over 500 enthusiastic teachers and role models to show a better way of life for at least 12,000 families. Supervision, training, and reinforcement of knowledge for the VMVs was ongoing. HSAs also continued to meet with the Village Health and Water Committees, setting mutually acceptable village goals for improved sanitation and better health.

The horticultural program developed over 100 "kitchen gardens" on both sides of the Shire River. These became a source of family and village nutrition, and some families developed a market for their carrots, tomatoes, green beans, sweet potatoes, cabbages, melons, and other produce. Perhaps one of the most valuable gardening efforts was the integration of the knowledge at the Standard Eight level of elementary school. There were two schools that added Gardening as a component of their curriculum. The children seemed to love the activity, for they not only prepared and planted their plots, they sold their plants, mature products and gathered seeds to plant the next season. They learned "hot-bed" systems for development of young plants to sell for home gardens, as well as transplanting into their larger garden. And the real pay-off of the school-based demonstration gardens was in the children learning to eat and enjoy their harvest and improve their dietary regimen. We had to assume that there was at least a bit of knowledge transfer from the children to their parents and even to grandparents!

Immunization Clinics were established in the 22 villages and the "cold chain" for keeping vaccines chilled with either dry ice or wet ice, from the time the supply left the Ministry of Health District refrigerators until they were administered appropriately at the village clinics. During these first two years of this Child Survival project, we built no clinic buildings. In some villages, space for weekly or monthly clinics was available at schools, churches and even at the village bar room. While mothers waited their turn for children's immunization or nutrition assessments, they were taught health messages by the HSAs or the VMVs.

Nutrition clinics were established by HSAs, sometimes jointly with the two Catholic Parish Clinics. Here, babies were weighed and measured and wherever malnutrition was detected, the baby was provided with enriched cereal formula and mothers were instructed in special feeding techniques. VMVs kept records for all babies who were failing to thrive and tracked the improvements over time.

Eleven new shallow wells were either completed as we described or were well on their way to completion, with a very responsible Malawian in charge of further development of ADRA supported clean water systems..

The CSAC continued its work but met less often, to guide the project and propose changes or expansions as appropriate. Because of this support, intergovernmental relationships were excellent. The support system of the other NGOs in Child Survival functioned for mutual support and accountability. Since ADRA does not employ Peace Corps Volunteers (PCVs) from the USA, we appreciated the working relationship that we developed with these energetic and well-prepared volunteers. PCV Cindy was attached to the Malawi Ministry of Health as a Health Educator for AIDS intervention. She provided us with posters and literature as well as condoms for distribution along with prevention education. John was assigned the Blantyre-based International Eye Foundation program and served as outreach worker assisting other NGOs in Nsanje and Chikwawa District. Sometimes Cindy or John traveled with us, or met us as we conducted village health committee meetings. There was a high degree of synergy in the total collaboration of many different agencies.

At least four drama teams were teaching and in demand in all the villages, especially for their *Edze* prevention themes. Some were able to travel by bus to teach and "entertain" entire neighboring villages.

In the project villages, a system for recording births and deaths was devised with the Village Chief or Headman appointing a member of the Health Committee to keep such records. Mid-way in our Malawi experience, we met one time with the national Director of Statistics who informed me that she would probably follow our model to develop the first national system for Vital Statistics. At that time, there were no funds to undertake such a venture and the Director of Statistics said she had hoped that ADRA would just take the lead in developing the national system. All I could do was just to smile.

In terms of financial accountability for the project, we never exceeded our budget, even though we could not account for $30,000.00. Our experience changed the worldwide accounting system for ADRA's relief and development operations.

The metaphor of "moonsmoke" no longer fit the improved picture of those villages where this "army" was deployed. With good leadership from among the HSAs and a new Project Manager from the U.S., the Nsanje District Child Survival Project had begun to lift the miasma of ignorance and disease wherever it had spread. The dispersal of that metaphorical putrid cloud of *moon smoke* seemed to us like the result of the gentle breeze of the active Spirit of Jesus Christ moving among these precious people.

EPILOGUE

AFTER GLOW

Ken and I readily admit that the nearly two years in Africa changed us a great deal. We often felt guilty at being blest with so much of God's goodness here in America, when there are so many millions of beautiful people living without education, without adequate food, clothing or shelter, and without a heart full of God's love and knowing nothing of the Christ Who loves them and wants to save them from their current condition. We had learned a new kind of patience with others. And we had a story to tell that we hoped would motivate those who heard the story to make a time in their lives when they will also volunteer for His service either in the ghettos of this nation or in one of the many third worlds, developing nations.

Four years after arriving home, I was invited to tell the story of the African women with whom I had worked during the annual Christian Women's Retreat in McCall, Idaho. Videos of the HSAs and Ngabu Dorika touched the hearts of nearly 200 women and a fire of self-sacrifice was lighted. These generous women sponsored a sewing machine project that ultimately placed four treadle machines, sewing notions and equipment, and 30 yards of fabric in those four separate villages in Malawi. In fact, when news spread to another group of women with great hearts, the Boise Quilters' Guild added money to make the project grow to serve the fourth village women's organization. You see, after we got home, Ken and I did provide a reconditioned sewing machine to the Dorika women at Ngabu through the help of our friend Hamed. This Income Generating Activity in Ngabu sparked enthusiasm with other women's groups across the entire lower Shire Valley.

By phone, I contacted Hamed, our Asian merchant-friend in Blantyre, again, to order the four machines. He was very willing to obtain the machines from a manufacturer in China, but he insisted that Ken and I must come back to Malawi to deliver the machines and supplies. The round trip tickets purchased privately at that time were $2500.00 each, and I told Hamed it was not possible for us to come. He insisted, saying "Mother, you and Father Ken must come and do this. My people in the Malawi bush trust you, but they need you there to celebrate with them, instruct them, and to pray with them." My heart thumped as I heard this precious Muslim man telling me that I needed to pray with these mostly Christian women! "Mother, you must come. You will stay in my home...You will drive my 4-wheel drive pick-up...You will spend at least a month enjoying Malawi, even staying in my cottage at the lake." Very much subdued and grateful, but having no idea how we could afford the trip, I promised Hamed that I would pray about what he said and see what God would show me. In my Malawi files, I found the FAX number for the Netherlands travel agency that is operated by those great Catholic women. It was an 800 number, so I sent our request for a "Least-Cost" price quote round trip to Malawi. The answer came back, $1500.00 each. So, after praying a few days, we decided that here was another opportunity to serve the people we love, and we drew from our retirement savings and made the trip.

By then, five years had elapsed, so we had to find a house and dog sitter and notify the recipient groups of the sewing IGA plan to help them get started with a program like that one in Ngabu. Numerous requests came in for us to bring good books, so we had several boxes of books for which British Airways charged no shipping all the way from Seattle to Blantyre. We spent a wonderful month being welcomed with singing and dancing in those four villages and visiting with many of the HSAs still active with their original villages, only now they were on the payroll of the Malawi Ministry of Health. Because we took that challenge, years earlier, when the Nsanje District Health Director told us we could not get to those remote villages, and we did it anyway – thousands of lives were changed. For us, this revisitation was like putting the frosting on the cake the Lord had helped us bake much earlier.

One of the pastor-leaders who helped us so much in the very early days of the project is Pastor Jim Nazombe. He had transferred from Nsanje District to Mwanza, an area near where he had grown up and where his parents still lived. The Dorika in Mwanza received one of the sewing machines with much pomp and ceremony. Just like the other three groups receiving this great start in earning power, they involved the rest of their church and shared their goals for use of the funds with us. Suddenly, during their ceremony of acceptance, one of the *bambos* entered the church where the ceremony was taking place with a huge stalk of bananas and placed them at our feet as a token of gratitude! The Dorika leader explained that we must take these bananas back to Idaho for the women who had sent the sewing machine! We bowed deeply to her and to the group and expressed appreciation on behalf of the women in Idaho. As we said goodbye, they loaded the bananas into Hamed's pickup, and for a while, we even thought we might find a shipper to fly them to Idaho, but it was not possible. So we took some of them to Hamed's family and the rest to Blantyre Adventist Hospital.

Pastor Jim Nazombe is still like a son to us, and we are pleased to report that by God's help we were able to sponsor him to four years of study at Solusi University in Zimbabwe where he recently completed a Bachelor of Arts degree, majoring in Theology. Of course, his appetite for education gives him a strong desire to attend graduate school at Solusi, but, for now, our Heavenly Father has called him back to teach and pastor in northern Malawi. Unless "Westerners" like us sponsor some of the best and brightest in countries like Malawi, higher education is out of their reach. It is our prayer that something in this book inspires you, dear reader, to invest in the preparation of messengers of the Good News of our Savior. We promise you and our God that proceeds from this book will help train more messengers to pick up the joyful responsibility!

~ THE END ~

Glossary of Terms

ADRA:	Adventist Development and Relief Agency
ADD:	Agricultural Development Director
Bambos:	Chichewa term for young men or fathers
Boma:	Community
Chabuka:	A powerful, village brew
Chadzuka bwanje:	"Good morning"
Chichewa:	The native language of Malawi

CSAC:	Child Survival Advisory Committee
Chitenji:	Chichewa article of clothing; also used as container tying up a load of goods for carrying on the head; also useful to tie baby on one's back
Dorika:	Chichewa term for Biblical person named, "Dorcas" who had a heart for helping the poor and those with special needs.
DIP:	Detailed Implementation Plan
Edze:	AIDS disease
HAS:	Health Surveillance Assistant, a mid-level village health worker as designated by the Malawi Ministry of Health
HI:	Health Inspector, a senior, professional community health leader
Izungu:	Chichewa for a white person
IGA:	Income generating activity
KAP:	Knowledge, Attitudes and Practices (as in a population study)

Katundu:	One's belongings, vernacular meaning is "stuff", as in "This is my stuff".
Kwacha:	The Malawi dollar, at that time the exchange rate was fourteen kwacha to one US dollar.
Khonde:	Sun room, often an entry way
Madze odzidzirwa:	Cold water
Malumba:	A hardwood tree, used for furniture building
Matola:	Pay for one's lift by a passing motorist or lorry
Mayi:	Mother
MCP:	Malawi Congress Party
MU:	Malawi University
Muli bwanji:	"Hello, how are you?" Chichewa greeting
Mulungu:	God
Mulungu akudalitseni:	God bless you!
Ndili bwino, zikomo:	"I am very well, thank you." Response to greeting of "Muli bwanji."
NGO:	Non-governmental Agency, in development work for Malawi

Nsima:	The standard mainstay in diet of Malawians, a thick paste of ground cooked maize meal.
Sena:	A dialect spoken in the southernmost part of Malawi, which seemed to be influenced greatly by the Portuguese spoken in neighboring Mozambique
SoBo:	Short term for Malawi Southern Bottling Co.
Tambala:	Chichewa for penny-type coin
UNICEF:	United Nations International Children's Educational Fund
USAID:	United States Agency for International Development
UNICEF:	United Nations International Children's Educational Fund
Zikomo:	A gracious greeting that means, "Thank you for coming", "You're welcome", or just and expression of deep appreciation, usually accompanied with gestures of hands together and a bow or curtsy.
Zungu:	Shortened Chichewa for white person

Breinigsville, PA USA
14 December 2010
251366BV00005B/12/A

9 781598 003420